50
SIMPLE
THINGS
YOU CAN
DO TO
SAVE YOUR
LIFE

FACULTY OF THE UCLA
SCHOOL OF PUBLIC HEALTH

Earthworks Press
Berkeley, California

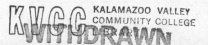

For Jesse. A long life.

THIS BOOK IS PRINTED ON RECYCLED PAPER

Created and Packaged by Javnarama
Designed by Javnarama
Cover Idea by Dayna Macy
Cover Art Direction by Sharon Smith
Cover Design by Madeline Budnick
Illustration by Robert Evans
ISBN 1-879682-11-7
First Edition 10 9 8 7 6 5 4 3 2 1

We've provided a great deal of information about
practices and products in this book. In most cases,
we've relied on advice, recommendations and research by
others whose judgments we consider accurate and free
from bias. However, we can't and don't guarantee
the results. This book offers you a start. The
responsibility for using it ultimately rests with you.

This book is intended as a reference volume only, not as
a medical manual. It is not a substitute for any treatment that
may have been prescribed by your doctor. If you suspect
that you have a medical problem, we urge you
to seek competent medical help.

For ordering information on
bulk rates and customized editions, write to
Earthworks Press
1400 Shattuck Avenue, #25
Berkeley, CA 94709

Distributor to the Book Trade: Publisher's Group West

ACKNOWLEDGMENTS

Thanks to all the people and organizations who worked with us to make this book possible, including:

Michael S. Goldstein, Ph. D.

John Javna

Mike Lynberg

Lynn Kebow

Fritz Springmeyer

Lyn Speakman

Melissa Schwarz

Sharilyn Hovind

Jack Mingo

Catherine Dee

Sharon Smith

Dayna Macy

Denise Silver

Jim Sanchirico

Melanie Foster

Nancy Skinner

Emma Lauriston

Lenna Lebovich

Ellen Umansky

John Dollison

Sven Newman

Joanne Miller

Randy Fleming

Ron Andersen, Ph.D.

Emil Berkanovic, Ph.D.

Linda Bourque, Ph.D.

Lester Breslow, M.D., M.P.H.

E. Richard Brown, Ph.D.

Climis Davos, Ph.D.

Roger Detels, M.D.

Pamela I. Erickson, M.P.H.

James Freed, D.D.S., M.P.H.

David Heber, M.D., Ph.D.

Inga Hoffman, M.P.H.

Derrick B. Jelliffe, M.D.

Alfred H. Katz, D.S.W., M.S.

Jess F. Kraus, Ph.D.

Peter A. Lachenbruch, Ph.D.

Roberta Malmgren, Ph.D.

Donald E. Morisky, Sc.D., M.S.P.H.

Alfred K. Neumann, M.D., M.P.H.

Mario Panaqua, B.A.

Shane Que Hee, Ph.D.

Susan C. M. Scrimshaw, Ph.D.

Judith M. Siegel, Ph.D.

Susan Sorenson, Ph.D.

Barbara Visscher, M.D., Dr. P.H.

Steven P. Wallace, Ph.D.

Tim Goodman

Dane Chapin

Mary Beth Train

Jennifer Chapin

Jeff Stafford

Nenelle Bunnin

Gordon Javna

CONTENTS

IT TAKES A COMMITMENT

Note: These subjects are listed in random order, not in order of importance.

INTRODUCTION

Hardly a day goes by when we don't hear about a study telling us how a certain diet, exercise program, or lifestyle will help us live longer and healthier lives. Clearly, if we do the "right things" we have more power over our health than was previously thought. But where do we start?

At the UCLA School of Public Health, our goals are disease prevention and health promotion. We conduct research on everything from AIDS, cancer, and aging to air pollution, health-care access, and the special problems of groups such as mothers, children, and minorities. But research is only half our job. The other half is education that leads to a healthier society, and that is why we wrote this book.

You will find no startling revelations in the pages ahead, no controversial assertions. What is new is that, for the first time, all of this information and advice is together in one resource—presented in the same readable fashion that EarthWorks Press popularized in the bestseller *50 Simple Things You Can Do to Save the Earth.*

No matter how easy this information is to follow, it is of little value unless it is used. *50 Simple Things You Can Do to Save Your Life* is an action manual. We present this book with the hope that you will not only learn something and use it for future reference, but also that you will be spurred to make the lifestyle changes that will improve your health and the health of those around you.

The health of those around you? Absolutely. Whether you're working to clean up the environment, to stop the spread of AIDS, or to reduce stress levels around you, your actions make a difference not only for your health, but for your community's. That's what public health—and this book—are all about.

Special credit for this project must go to Dr. Michael Goldstein, who helped conceptualize it and coordinated the efforts of the faculty; and John Javna, Michael Lynberg and Lynn Kebow. Without these four individuals, the book would not exist.

Here's to your good health.

—*Abdelmonem A. Afifi, Ph.D.*
Dean, UCLA School of Public Health

SIMPLE

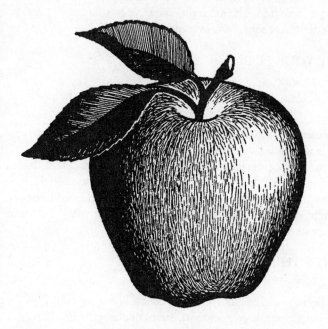

THINGS

1. FIND YOUR ROOTS

Almost 1/3 of all known diseases and conditions are linked to heredity.

What difference does it make to your health if your aunt had cancer...Or if your great-grandfather had heart trouble? Maybe none at all; but it could mean that you're likely to get them, too. The more you know about your family history, the better chance you have of protecting yourself.

SAVE YOUR LIFE

• If you know you're at risk for a disease because of heredity, you can do a lot to prevent it—either by changing your habits, or by staying vigilant and detecting problems early.

• For example: Comedian Gilda Radner died of ovarian cancer, a disease with as much as an 85% survival rate if it's caught early. She and her doctors didn't realize that her aunt, first cousin, and probably her grandmother had suffered from the disease—which raised her risk from the usual 1-in-70 to 1-in-2. If they had, they would have been on the lookout for it, and might have caught it in time to save her life.

SIMPLE THINGS YOU CAN DO

1. Know Your Risk

• Collect as much medical data as possible about your family—great-grandparents, grandparents, aunts, uncles, parents, siblings, and children.

• The best sources of this information are members of your family. You can also check doctors' records, hospital records, or even state death certificates. However, medical records regarding cause of death are often unreliable or hard to decipher.

2. Know What to Look For

• Find out about all major diseases, surgeries, and causes of death. (You may also want to include chronic ailments like ulcers.) If complete information isn't available, at least try to find out how people died and how old they were at the time. Any data will help.

- Pay attention to your parents' dependencies, including prescription and over-the-counter drugs.

- Find out *when* your relatives had their heart attacks and strokes. The earlier the heart attack, the greater the chance the disease is genetic. (Note: If the victim smoked, you can add ten years to their age.) A long-term study in Massachusetts has demonstrated that people whose parents or siblings had heart attacks before age 60 have twice the risk for early coronaries.

- Look for patterns in the types of cancers your family has had. It may mean you're at risk for developing the same kind of cancer…at a younger than average age. For instance, "In families with many cases of colon cancer," says cancer specialist Henry Lynch, "the condition hits at an average age of 44 years—instead of the more typical 60 or 65. Hereditary breast cancer comes on at an average age of 42 instead of 63."

- Other diseases that may run in families include psychological disorders (like "manic depression"), alcoholism, depression, schizophrenia, asthma, arthritis, and gall bladder disease.

3. Plan Ahead

- To keep this information organized, put together a *genogram*—a family tree that lists your close relatives' major physical and mental problems.

- List your immediate relatives. Fill in their names, dates of birth and death, and marriage information. Beside each one, list major illness, cause of death, and how old they were.

- Give a copy to your doctor and discuss any hereditary diseases and how you can prevent them. Tell your doctor about your family's chemical dependency history before he or she prescribes drugs to you.

- Keep your genogram current so your children and other family members will be able to use it later.

RESOURCES

- *Discover Your Roots: A New, Easy Guide for Tracing Your Family Tree.* By Marilyn M. Heimberg (Communication Creativity, 1977). $3.95. *Check for it at your local bookstore.*

2. AN APPLE A DAY

*Studies have found a lower incidence of colon and rectal
cancer in people who frequently eat cabbage.*

Your parents were right about at least one thing, anyway—it
really *is* important to eat your fruits and vegetables. Fruits
and vegetables help lower the risk of potentially fatal illnesses like heart disease and some cancers...yet 90% of Americans
eat only half the amount recommended by the FDA.

EAT FOR LIFE

• Fruits and vegetables that contain vitamin C (berries, melons,
etc.) are believed to help prevent pancreatic and colon cancer.

• Cruciferous vegetables (broccoli, cabbage, brussels sprouts, cauli-
flower, kohlrabi, and kale) have been linked to lower rates of colon
cancer, lung cancer, and skin tumors.

• Deep-orange and dark-green vegetables (carrots, spinach, kale,
squash, sweet potatoes) are believed to help prevent cancer of the
lungs, mouth, colon, breast, and larynx, because they contain beta-
carotene, which our bodies turn into vitamin A.

• Fruits and vegetables are a good source of fiber, which moves
food—and potential carcinogens—out of the body. (See p. 37)

SIMPLE THINGS YOU CAN DO

1. Know What to Look For

• Consult a nutritional guide (see p. 33) and find out which fruits
and vegetables provide the nutrients you need. For example: Peach-
es, bananas, and watermelons contain carotene. Spinach and avo-
cadoes contain vitamin C. Dried fruits like raisins, dates, prunes,
and dried apricots are good sources of iron and potassium.

2. Eat More Fruits and Vegetables

• Experts recommend at least 5 servings of fruit and vegetables
every day. That sounds like a lot, but it's not. One serving equals
1/2 cup of fruit or cooked vegetables, 1 cup of leafy vegetables, or
1/4 cup of dried fruit.

3. CARRY A MEDICAL ID

Americans visit hospital emergency rooms 77 million times every year.

I magine you've been knocked unconscious in an accident. You're taken to a hospital emergency room, but you can't tell doctors that you have a medical condition—like an allergy to penicillin—that requires special attention.

How can you protect yourself in this potentially life-threatening situation? Wear or carry a medical ID.

SIMPLE THINGS YOU CAN DO

1. Know Your Risk

• According to Medic Alert, "one in five Americans has a medical condition that places them at added risk in an emergency."

• These conditions include diabetes, heart trouble, epilepsy, hemophilia, allergies, and possibly even wearing contact lenses, if the patient is unconscious.

2. Protect Yourself

• Carry a medical ID card. You can make your own and carry it in your wallet. Include your name, address, phone number, the person to call in an emergency, your doctor's name and phone number, blood type, any allergies (to drugs, insect bites, etc.), medical conditions, and any required medications.

• Wear a medical ID necklace or bracelet. It may be better than a card, since it's more easily noticed in an emergency. Ask your doctor where to get one.

• Join Medic Alert. This nonprofit group offers the most comprehensive emergency service available. They supply a bracelet or necklace, and a wallet ID card. They also have a toll-free, 24-hour emergency phone hotline that can provide hospitals with your complete medical history—including names of doctors and family members to contact. Cost is $35 for a lifetime membership, $7 to update records. Call 1-800-ID-ALERT for more information.

4. LEARN THE HEIMLICH MANEUVER

Each year, 2,500 to 4,000 people choke to death. Many could be saved with this simple technique.

Brent Meldrum was only 5 years old when his neighbor, Tanya Branden (age 6), began choking on a piece of candy.

"My mother was screaming at me to get away from her, but I knew what to do," Brent recalls. He'd recently seen the technique demonstrated on one of his favorite TV shows.

Brent put his arms around Tanya from behind—she was now turning blue—clasped his hands together, and squeezed, lifting the girl off the floor. "I banged her feet down on the floor, and she bended over and coughed, and it plopped out."

Brent saved a life. And you can, too, if you learn the Heimlich maneuver. It takes only a few minutes.

BREATHTAKING FACTS

• Choking occurs when food or some other object slips into a person's trachea (or airway) instead of into the esophagus (the tube next to the airway that leads to the stomach). This obstruction triggers a muscle spasm. The person can't breathe and chokes.

• In 1974, Dr. Henry Heimlich developed a revolutionary technique to save choking people. He found that a substantial amount of air is still left in the lungs when a person chokes—so if a fist is pressed into a choking person's abdomen and thrust upward, the force of the air can literally pop an obstruction out of the throat and mouth.

• According to Dr. Heimlich: "The maneuver avoids the problems with past approaches to handling choking. Inserting a finger or other object to retrieve an obstructing piece of food or other item risks driving it farther down. Pounding on the back is inherently dangerous because it may wedge the material more deeply."

SIMPLE THINGS YOU CAN DO

1. Know Your Risk

• Adults have a higher risk of choking when they drink alcohol while eating, eat in a hurry, or laugh hard while eating.

• Children often choke if they have food in their mouths while they're doing something else, like running or playing.

2. Know What to Look For

• If someone can't talk and grabs their throat, that person may be choking. You only have about 4 minutes to respond. After this, the lack of oxygen can cause permanent brain damage or death.

3. Use the Heimlich Maneuver

Note: It's possible to hurt someone with this maneuver—and special techniques are called for with young children, unconscious people, or while performing it on yourself. We recommend learning from a class (it's taught in CPR classes), illustrated guide, or video. In the meantime, here's a basic description of the technique:

• Quickly stand behind the victim and wrap your arms around the waist.

• Make a fist and place the thumb side against the victim's abdomen, slightly above the belly button and below the rib cage.

• Grab your fist with your other hand and give three or four quick, upward thrusts. Note: Simply squeezing won't do the trick—you have to use enough force so that air from the lungs dislodges whatever is stuck in the windpipe.

• If at first you don't succeed, try again—several times if necessary.

RESOURCES

Most first-aid books have illustrated instructions. Or try one of these:

• **Dr. Heimlich's Home First Aid Video**, produced by MCA Home Video. *Features Dr. Heimlich demonstrating a number of life-saving techniques. Check your local video store.*

• **First Aid for Choking Wall Chart.** *Charts for performing the maneuver on adults, children, or infants, 25¢ each. Contact your local American Heart Association.*

5. CHECK YOUR BLOOD PRESSURE

*It's estimated that as many as 15 million Americans
have high blood pressure...without knowing it.*

Y ou're not tense, nervous, or jumpy...and you feel fine. So you
couldn't have high blood pressure...right?
Wrong. Normally, there are no noticeable symptoms of
high blood pressure (or "hypertension")—despite the fact that it is
a major cause of both heart disease and stroke.

High blood pressure is usually controllable with lifestyle changes
and medication. But if it's left untreated, your chance of dying before the age of 65 is two to three times higher than that of a person
with normal blood pressure.

That's why it's important to get your blood pressure checked
regularly. The test is painless and simple, it only takes a few
minutes...and it may save your life.

BLOOD PRESSURE BASICS

What is blood pressure, anyway?

• The American Heart Association explains it this way: "The beating of your heart pumps blood through large blood vessels called arteries; they conduct blood from your heart to other parts of your
body. As your blood is pumped through your arteries, it pushes
against the arterial walls. This force against the walls of the arteries
is called blood pressure."

What is *high* blood pressure?

• Arteries consist of three layers; the second layer is muscular.

• When the muscular layer contracts, an artery gets smaller. It becomes like a four-lane freeway that's narrowed to two lanes: The
heart is pumping the same amount of blood, but there's not as
much room for it. Result: Too much pressure on the artery walls.

• In some people, the arterial muscles contract permanently.
That's chronic high blood pressure; no one's sure what causes it.

SIMPLE THINGS YOU CAN DO

1. Know Your Risk

• Contrary to common belief, high blood pressure isn't necessarily caused by stress. In fact, according to the American Heart Association, "about 90% of all cases of high blood pressure have no known cause."

• More men develop high blood pressure than women.

• In men, the majority of cases develop between the ages of 30 and 45; women seem to develop it later, after menopause. Some serious cases begin even earlier, during childhood.

• African-Americans are twice as likely to have it as Caucasians and often get it more severely. No one's sure why.

• If your parents had it, you're more likely to have it.

• Substantially overweight people are more likely to develop it.

2. Get Tested

• Have your blood pressure checked at least once a year. Your doctor will usually take your blood pressure during an annual exam. If you just want your blood pressure checked, call the American Red Cross (many local chapters offer free screenings), the American Heart Association (provides referrals for local tests), or your local fire department (many offer blood pressure tests).

• Several things can elevate blood pressure temporarily. If you drink a lot of coffee, eat a large meal, exert yourself physically, or smoke a few cigarettes before getting your blood pressure checked, it can register higher than normal. Even simple nervousness can raise blood pressure. Some people get so tense at a doctor's office that their blood pressure skyrockets.

• If you test high, get two more tests. If all three tests register high, see a doctor. A lifestyle change is usually the first prescription. Most cases can be controlled by reducing weight, getting aerobic exercise, cutting down on salt and caffeine, quitting smoking, and managing stress. If these measures don't work, the doctor will probably prescribe medication.

RESOURCE

• **The National Hypertension Association,** 324 East 30th St., New York, NY 10016; (212) 889-3557. *Write or call for information.*

6. GET IMMUNIZED

*Although adults can die from tetanus, nearly half of
American adults aren't up to date on their booster shots.*

If you've had the standard childhood immunizations, you probably think you've had all the shots you need. Right? Well, you may need a few more. There are at least seven serious diseases for which adult immunization is commonly recommended: influenza, measles, rubella, hepatitis B, tetanus, diphtheria, and pneumococcal infections.

SIMPLE THINGS YOU CAN DO

1. Know Your Risk

• If you were vaccinated for measles between 1957 and 1967, you may need another vaccination; the vaccine may have been ineffective. If you haven't had the measles or any vaccination, you may need to be immunized. Check with your doctor.

• Hepatitis B is a sexually transmitted disease. If you're sexually active, you should get immunized. The vaccine is generally considered safe for everyone, but according to one expert, "Less than one quarter of high-risk people have been vaccinated."

• Hepatitis B can also be transmitted by coming into contact with an infected person's blood. So vaccination is recommended for certain high-risk groups, such as medical and dental personnel.

• Annual flu shots are recommended for people over 65, anyone with diseases of the heart, liver or kidneys, diabetes, asthma, or any lung disorder. It's also recommended for health-care workers, cancer patients who are under treatment, and any person with AIDS—or whose immune system is suppressed for any reason.

• Flu shots are not recommended for healthy adults under 65, since influenza is almost never fatal for them. It's also not recommended for people sensitive to eggs or egg products, as the shot can give them a severe allergic reaction. If you're pregnant, wait until after your third month before you're vaccinated.

• About 40 million people should get flu shots every year, but only about 20% of those at risk do. One result: According the Centers for Disease Control, in the flu outbreak of 1989-90 an estimated 58,000 Americans died.

• Flu season in the U.S. usually takes place between December and March. Doctors recommend getting vaccinated in early November because it takes about two weeks for the body to build up its immunity.

• The same groups who should be immunized for the flu should be vaccinated for pneumococcal pneumonia—but just once. Repeat booster shots are not recommended except in very special cases.

• There are an estimated 250,000 to 500,000 cases of pneumococcal pneumonia every year in the U.S. About 40,000 deaths result, despite the fact that many are preventable with the vaccine.

• It's recommended that everyone get a diphtheria and tetanus booster every 10 years. People associate tetanus with deep puncture wounds (such as that caused by stepping on a nail), but there have been cases of tetanus resulting from something as minor as pricking a finger on a rose thorn or getting scratched in the garden.

2. Protect Yourself

• Review your immunization history to find out if you need a vaccination. If you haven't kept records, contact your family doctor. If in doubt, the safest bet is to assume you haven't been immunized. Consult your doctor about the appropriate vaccine.

• If you don't have a physician, call your local public health department for vaccine information. They often have supplies of vaccines on hand and may even give shots free.

3. Plan Ahead

• Get an official state immunization record form from your city or county health department. Take it with you to every medical checkup (yours and your children's) so doctors can record each vaccine dose as it is given, along with the date.

7. GET A PAP SMEAR

*An estimated 4,500 woman die of cervical cancer each year. If all women
had regular Pap smears, nine out of ten of these lives could be saved.*

The Pap smear is a simple exam that can help you tell whether you have cervical cancer...or a condition that might lead to it.

Do you have a Pap smear regularly? There's really no reason to put it off. At worst, the test may be a little uncomfortable...but it can save your life.

SAVE YOUR LIFE

• According to the National Cancer Institute, cervical cancer is now almost 100% curable if diagnosed early and treated promptly.

• The Pap smear is particularly important because cervical cancer usually has no symptoms in its early stages.

• Since the Pap smear was introduced, 70% fewer women die from cervical cancer.

SIMPLE THINGS YOU CAN DO

1. Know Your Risk

• Cervical cancer is most likely to occur in women between the ages of 30 and 55.

• Women who smoke are 3 times as likely to develop cervical cancer as nonsmokers.

• Women who began having sexual intercourse before age 18 and women who have had many sex partners have an increased risk of developing cervical cancer.

• Women whose mothers were given the drug *diethylstilbestrol* (DES) during pregnancy to prevent miscarriage are also at risk.

• Some researchers believe the sexually transmitted viruses that cause genital warts—and perhaps those that cause genital herpes—may also cause cervical cancer. That may put women who've contracted these conditions at added risk.

2. Get Tested

• If you're over 18, or you've had sexual intercourse, an annual pelvic exam and Pap smear are recommended. This is especially important if you're at high risk for cervical cancer.

• Pap smears can be performed less frequently if you have three or more normal annual exams because cervical cancer develops slowly. Discuss it with your doctor.

• According to many sources, the best time to have a Pap smear is 2 weeks after the first day of the last menstrual period. To get the most accurate results, don't have intercourse for 24 hours prior to the test, and avoid douching and vaginal contraceptives for 72 hours before the test.

3. Protect Yourself

• According to the American College of Obstetricians and Gynecologists, signs of trouble may be missed in up to 40% of women with precancerous or cancerous conditions.

• The accuracy of this test depends on a number of factors, including the doctor's sampling technique and how carefully the slide that contains the sample is prepared, transported, and stored.

• To improve the chances of accuracy:

√ Find out about the lab that will process your test. It should be accredited by either the College of American Pathologists or the American Society of Cytology.

√ Find out if the lab provides a full written report.

√ Ask your doctor to let you know your results, even if they're normal. If you haven't heard anything in three weeks, call.

• If you're in a high-risk group, consider having a second Pap test to confirm a negative result. If you're interested in other tests that may help detect cervical cancer, like *cervigrams*, ask your doctor.

• If your test is positive, don't panic. An abnormal Pap test does not necessarily mean you have cancer. It simply shows a need for further tests. In some cases it may indicate something as benign as a vaginal infection.

RESOURCES

• National Cancer Institute; (800) 4-CANCER. *Call for free brochure, "What You Need To Know About Cancer of the Cervix."*

8. STAY ACTIVE

*Mowing your lawn with a manual mower burns about 450
calories an hour—the same as an hour of tennis.*

Will weeding in your garden, dancing, or walking up a few
flights of stairs really help keep you healthy?
Numerous studies indicate that even small amounts of
physical activity can improve your health, help you stay slim, and
reduce your risk of heart attacks.

SIMPLE THINGS YOU CAN DO

1. Start Today.

• Walk or bicycle on some of your errands, instead of driving.

• When you go shopping, park a distance from the store and walk
to your destination. If you use public transportation, get off a few
stops early and walk the rest of the way.

• Use your shopping trips for exercise. If you're just buying a few
items in the grocery store, carry your selections instead of pushing a
shopping cart.

• Take the stairs instead of elevators and escalators.

• Go for a walk during your coffee breaks.

2. Plan Ahead

• Find ways to turn sedentary activity into physical activity. For
example, don't just read the paper or watch TV—peddle a station-
ary bike or do some sit-ups at the same time.

• Take a look around your home: What power machines can you
do without? You can get an easy workout from mowing the lawn,
sawing, digging, hand-mixing food, kneading bread, and other
household chores when you power them with your own muscles.

• Take up active hobbies. In an hour of gardening, for example,
you can burn 240-300 calories; bicycling uses 400-700 calories.

• When you're ready for a regular exercise program, see pages 24
and 38.

9. EARLY WARNING SYSTEM

Fifty percent of all cancer cases could be prevented with present knowledge.

People don't like to talk about cancer; we find it frightening. But the more each of us knows, the greater chance we have of preventing—or surviving—the disease. Learning the American Cancer Society's Seven Warning Signs is a good place to start.

SAVE YOUR LIFE
• One-third of all Americans—including children—will get some form of cancer in their lifetime.

• Cancer isn't necessarily fatal. There are over 7 million Americans alive today with a history of the disease. The key is early detection. As soon as a diagnosis is made, treatment can begin.

SIMPLE THINGS YOU CAN DO

Know What to Look For
• Learn the most common warning signs of cancer:
  C = Change in bowel or bladder habits
  A = A sore or scab that refuses to heal
  U = Unusual bleeding or discharge
  T = Thickening or lump in breast or elsewhere
  I = Indigestion or difficulty swallowing
  O = Obvious change in wart or mole
  N = Nagging cough or hoarseness

• Don't wait for symptoms to become uncomfortable or painful; pain isn't usually an early symptom of cancer.

• These symptoms can be caused by problems besides cancer. However, it's important to see a doctor if any symptom lasts as long as 2 weeks. For more info, call the American Cancer Society (1-800-ACS-2345) or National Cancer Institute (1-800-4-CANCER).

10. BUCKLE UP

*According to the U.S. Department of Transportation, you have a
1-in-3 chance of being in a serious car accident sometime in your life.*

Nancy Skinner was four blocks from home when her car was
hit by a driver who'd run a stop sign. The force of the impact pushed her vehicle off the road, and it careened down
the sidewalk, hitting a concrete bench, a tree, a sign, and finally a
retaining wall.

If Nancy and her daughter hadn't been wearing their seatbelts,
they would have been thrown in a different direction with each impact. Fortunately, their seatbelts were buckled. "It was a simple
shopping trip I make every day," Nancy says. "It never seemed
there was any risk involved. I used to be a casual seatbelt user; now
I'm a fanatic. There's no question that seatbelts save lives."

SAVE YOUR LIFE

• More than half the people killed in passenger car crashes could
be saved if all occupants wore their seatbelts. Yet a majority of drivers and passengers (53%) still don't wear them.

• Some people feel seatbelts aren't worth the trouble on short
drives. But 75% of all accidents occur within 25 miles of home.

• Others think they're safe at slower speeds. But 8 of 10 fatal crashes happen under 40 mph.

• Many people think they won't get hurt if they brace themselves
during a crash. But the impact is over in 1/10 of a second...and it's
powerful: In a 30-mph collision with a solid object, for example, an
unbelted passenger will hit the windshield (or other object) with a
force equal to jumping head first from a 5-story building.

• Some drivers don't wear seatbelts because they think it's safer to
be thrown clear of an accident. But it's not. Studies show you are
25-40 times more likely to be killed if you're thrown from a vehicle.

• Other drivers worry they may be trapped by seatbelts if a car is on
fire or underwater. But studies show that chances of survival are actually *greater* with a seatbelt on, because people are less likely to be
knocked unconscious and can escape.

SIMPLE THINGS YOU CAN DO

1. Protect Yourself

• Wear your seatbelt...and insist your passengers wear one, too.

• If you own a used car that doesn't have safety belts, go to a dealer and have them installed.

• A lap belt should be low on your hips. This reduces chance or severity of injury by spreading impact over the stronger hip bones.

• Don't wear a shoulder belt without a lap belt. If you slide forward in an accident, it may strangle you. Now that new cars are equipped with automatic shoulder belts, this is important.

• Don't rely on airbags alone. They'll protect you in a head-on crash, but may not protect you if you're hit on the side, are rear-ended, or if your car flips over.

2. Protect Your Children

• A child held in your lap won't be safe in a crash. If you're not wearing a seatbelt, you can crush the child against the dashboard. If you are wearing one, the child can fly from your arms with the force of thousands of pounds.

• Children under 4 years of age (about 40 lbs.) should ride in child safety seats that meet all federal safety standards. But follow the instructions. According to the National Safety Council, "an estimated 70% of the children who die each year in car accidents would survive if parents used child safety seats correctly and consistently."

• The major cause of death for pregnant women is auto accidents. Many pregnant women don't wear seatbelts—they worry that the belt will hurt the fetus in an accident. It won't. In nearly 100% of crashes, the fetus recovers quickly from any pressure a seatbelt exerts and suffers no lasting injury.

RESOURCES

• Contact your local AAA office about safety belt information, including "Safety Belt Use Required" decals.

National Safety Council, 444 North Michigan Ave., Chicago, IL 60611; (312)527-4800. *Send for pamphlets "Stay Alive and Stay Well" and "Ride 'em Safely!" (on proper use of child safety seats).*

11. AEROBIC EXERCISE

*Three 20-30 minute aerobic workouts a week is a big start
toward healthier heart, lungs, bones and muscles.*

Y ou don't need a lot of exercise to keep fit—experts say three
20-30 minute *vigorous* aerobic workouts or three 40-60 minute *moderate* aerobic workouts each week will do it.

Think about that—a few hours a week may be all it takes to dra-
matically reduce your risk of getting heart disease, strokes and some
types of cancer. Despite this, fewer than 10% of American adults
exercise regularly.

Time to get started? The trick is finding the right aerobic exercise for you...and then making it a regular part of your life.

AEROBIC EXERCISE

• Aerobic literally means "with air." When you exercise, it means
your heart and lungs are using oxygen as efficiently as possible,
strengthening your cardiovascular system.

• Of course, the more strenuous the activity, the more calories you
burn. But what's important in aerobic exercise is is *how long* and
how often you do it—not how hard.

SIMPLE THINGS YOU CAN DO

1. Know What to Look For

• The secret to getting benefits from aerobic exercise is knowing
when your heart and lungs are working at optimum efficiency—not
too fast or too slow. (It's common for people to push too hard in
the beginning...and then give up altogether.)

• The way to tell if you're getting maximum benefit from your exercising is to calculate the "target heart rate" for your age. Then as
you exercise, check your pulse periodically and try to stay within
the target heart rate. Here's how to calculate your rate:

√ Start with the number 220.

√ Subtract your age from it.

√ Multiply that total first by 60%, and then 80%.

√ Your heartbeat rate per minute should fall between those two numbers as you exercise. (For example, if you're 40, your target rate is between 108 and 144 beats per minute).

√ During exercise, find a pulse point (on your wrist or neck).

√ Using a watch with a second hand, count your heartbeats for 6 seconds. Multiply by 10. If your heartbeat is below your target heart rate, speed up; if it's over your rate, slow down.

2. Protect Yourself

• Start and end your exercise slow and easy. Don't put on your shoes and dart out the door—your body likes it best if you start slowly for five minutes or so to get the blood flowing and the muscles warmed up. (This isn't considered part of your workout.)

• *After* your warm-up, stretch your muscles gently and without pain—don't jerk or bounce as you stretch.

• At the end of your workout, slow down gradually for a few minutes to help prevent an abrupt drop in blood pressure and reduce muscle stiffness later.

• On a hot day your body can easily sweat out a quart of water an hour, so drink plenty of fluids.

3. Plan Ahead

• To maintain the benefits of exercise, you have to keep doing it. A recent study found that professional athletes who became sedentary eventually sank to the same conditioning level as people who had never exercised at all. On the other hand, starting now with a regular program, even if you've never exercised before, will start giving you immediate benefits.

RESOURCES

American College of Sports Medicine, PO Box 1440, Indianapolis, IN 46206-1440; (317) 637-9200. *Offers several brochures including* Achieving and Maintaining Physical Fitness. *Send a business-size SASE and $2.00 for a copy.*

• The President's Council on Physical Fitness and Sports, Superintendent of Documents, Government Printing Office, Washington, DC 20402-9325. *Has a list of good publications on fitness.*

12. PREVENT STDS

One out of every four Americans between the ages of 15 and 55 will catch at least one sexually transmitted disease sometime in their lives.

What are the most common infectious diseases in the U.S.? Colds, flu...and sexually transmitted diseases (STDs). More than 10 million Americans—nearly one-third of them teenagers—get STDs every year.

A lot of progress has been made in detecting and treating these diseases, but prevention is still the best—and surest—cure.

SAVE YOUR LIFE

• There are more than 30 different STDs. Many are rampant in America. Most can be successfully treated. (AIDS is one notable exception.) But because there are often no symptoms, many people with STDs don't realize they have them...and never get treatment.

• If chlamydia, the most common STD in the U.S. (3 to 4 million new cases a year), is left untreated, it can cause painful infections and infertility.

• Genital herpes has been linked with an increased risk of cervical cancer in women, and can be passed to an infant at childbirth. There are about 500,000 new U.S. cases each year.

• Gonorrhea is a bacterial infection that, if left untreated, can cause arthritis, reproductive problems, or even heart disease. There are as many as 2 million new cases a year in the U.S.

• Syphilis is now at a 40-year high; about 100,000 new cases are reported each year. If left untreated, it can cause permanent disability ...or death.

SIMPLE THINGS YOU CAN DO

1. Know Your Risk

• If you're in a monogamous relationship, if you and your partner test negative for STDs and don't use IV drugs, there's nothing to worry about. You're not at risk.

• If you have sex with more than one person, or your partner does, then you're at risk.

2. Know What to Look For

• Unfortunately, the most common symptom of an STD is no symptom at all.

• Symptoms that may appear include: an open sore or blister in the genital area, an unusual discharge, or an itching or burning sensation while urinating.

• A person with syphilis might experience swollen lymph nodes and flu-like symptoms about 6-8 weeks after exposure.

3. Protect Yourself

• Abstinence is your best protection.

• If you're sexually active, use a condom. Latex—not animal membrane or "skin"—condoms are the best protection against most STDs. Cervical caps and IUDs *will not* protect you.

• Use water-based lubricants (like K-Y Jelly) with condoms—*not* petroleum-based lubricants (Vaseline, baby oil), which can make latex condoms break apart. Try a lubricant with nonoxynol-9 for extra protection.

• For more protection, use birth control foam, cream or jelly with the condom. The chemicals in them kill many STD germs.

• If you have sex with more than one person, or your partner does, it's a good idea to get checked for STDs about once a year—even if you have no symptoms. Pregnant women should also get tests.

• Watch for signs of an STD in yourself and in your partner. If you have an STD, tell your sexual partner(s) so they can get tested. They may have it, too…which means they can be spreading the disease—and could even give it back to you.

• For more information on AIDS, see P. 40.

RESOURCES

• **The American Social Health Organization;** (800) 227-8922. *Call for info about doctors and clinics in your area that treat STDs.*

• **Planned Parenthood,** 810 Seventh Ave., New York, NY 10019. *Offers a variety of pamphlets on STDs and safe sex. Single copies are 75¢. Write for a free catalog.*

• **Do It Now Foundation,** 6423 South Ash Ave., Tempe, AZ 85283. *Write for free single copies of STD Blues and Safe Sex.*

13. BE PREPARED

In the next 12 months, one in four American children will suffer an injury serious enough to require medical attention.

Would you know who to call in a medical emergency? Do you know the quickest route from your house to the nearest hospital? Could an ambulance find your home easily? Being prepared for an emergency is one of the simplest...and most important...ways to protect yourself and your family.

SIMPLE THINGS YOU CAN DO

Plan Ahead

• Put a list of emergency phone numbers next to your phone, or in a prominent place near the phone. Include:

√ Police and fire departments

√ Hospitals

√ Ambulance services

√ The local poison control center.

√ Family doctors

√ Next-door neighbors and relatives to contact in an emergency.

• Teach your children the emergency phone number in your area (it's usually 911, but not in all communities) and how to give directions to your home.

• Locate the nearest hospital emergency room. Make a few practice runs, so you'll know the best route in an emergency. Leave a map of the route to the hospital in your car or by the phone.

• Make sure your street address is visible from the road (even at night) in case an ambulance needs to find it. Use large, reflective numbers, or make sure numbers are illuminated by porch or street lights.

• Make sure baby sitters understand your emergency phone list, know where to find fire extinguishers and first-aid kits, and know where you can be reached whenever you go out.

• Get and sign a consent form authorizing medical treatment in your absence from your local hospital. Leave it in a special place at home in case you can't be reached.

14. WALK RIGHT AT NIGHT

*Every year, about 3,500 pedestrians are hit
and killed by motor vehicles after dark.*

Remember when your parents and teachers used to tell you to "Walk on the green, not in between," "Look both ways before crossing," "Stop, look, and listen," and so on? How about "Wear white at night"?

Night is the most dangerous time to be walking. Fifty percent of all pedestrian deaths occur at night, even though there are fewer people on the streets then. Taking a few precautions may save your life.

SIMPLE THINGS YOU CAN DO

Protect Yourself

• If you're walking or jogging at night, wearing light-colored clothing makes it easier for drivers to see you...but it still may not be enough to protect you. Experts say that alert drivers, traveling at 40 mph, need at least 150 feet to stop. A pedestrian wearing a white shirt and jeans is visible at a distance of only about 200 feet—which may not give an average driver enough time to swerve or stop.

• Wear "reflectorized" material. Studies show that even when it's worn on dark clothing, this material enables a driver to see you as much as 750 feet sooner than normal. You can get reflectorized armbands, hats, headbands, patches, and even adhesive strips for your shoes at sporting good stores or toy stores. This is essential for people who jog at night.

• Your best bet if you're walking at night is to bring a flashlight. A pedestrian with a flashlight is visible 600 feet farther away than someone wearing reflective material.

• Don't "walk under the influence." It may sound silly, but about 35% of all pedestrian fatalities are people who've been drinking.

15. BREAST EXAM

*Recent studies show that only 25% of American women
perform routine breast self-exams every month.*

A question for women: What can you do that takes just a few
minutes a month...and could save your life?
Answer: A simple self-exam for breast cancer. Along
with getting a mammogram regularly, it's the best defense you've
got against this dangerous disease.

SAVE YOUR LIFE
• About 1 of every 9 women in the U.S. will develop breast cancer
in her lifetime. The American Cancer Society estimates that in a
single year 175,000 women develop it...and 44,500 die from it.
• However, if breast cancer is diagnosed and treated early enough,
the five-year survival rate is more than 90%.
• Mammograms (X-rays that use low levels of radiation to look
through a breast) can detect 80-90% of breast cancers, often years
before they can be felt in an exam. They can pick up a cancer the
size of a matchhead when chance of longterm survival is 90-98%.
However, over half of U.S. women over 40 say they haven't had a
mammogram...and 17% say they don't even know what it is.
• Self-exams are a vital part of diagnosis. About 90% of all breast
cancers are found by women themselves—not their doctors.

SIMPLE THINGS YOU CAN DO

1. Know Your Risk
• 75% of all breast cancer is found in women age 50 or older.
• A woman whose mother, sister, or daughter has had breast cancer is two to three times more likely to develop it herself. About
15% of breast cancers are hereditary.
• If you started menstruation at an early age (before age 11 or 12),
had a late menopause, had your first child after turning 30, or never
had children at all you're in the high-risk group.
• After menopause, a woman whose fat is concentrated in the abdomen may be more likely to develop breast cancer. One study

showed that a woman with a 39-inch waist is twice as likely to get it as a woman with a 32-inch waist, even if they weigh the same.

• However, bout 80% of women diagnosed with breast cancer have no risk factors at all.

2. Get Regular Mammograms

• Experts recommend that all women get a "baseline" mammogram between ages 35-40. This sets up a norm to compare to later. High-risk women should check with doctors about when to start.

• Women 40-50 years old should get mammograms every 1-2 years. After age 50, women should get one every year.

• Don't let the negative results of a mammogram make you careless. You still need to do self-exams, and continue to get mammograms.

3. Do Self-Exams

• Women over 18 should conduct a monthly self-exam for lumps. Schedule a lesson with your doctor or local clinic.

• In a recent survey, only 8% of the women performed self-exams correctly. Most of those who did had been trained by a doctor or nurse. Women who only learned from pamphlets did much worse. The biggest problem: They didn't look for lumps under their arms, where there's also breast tissue.

• If you find a lump, don't panic—80% of them are benign. But any lump that doesn't go away after a menstrual period should be checked by a doctor.

• Other symptoms to look for: a change in the size or shape of a breast; a discharge from a nipple; a change in the color or feel of the skin of a breast or aureola. They should be checked by a doctor.

RESOURCES

• National Alliance of Breast Cancer Organizations (NABCO), 1180 Avenue of the Americas, 2nd floor, New York, NY 10036; (212) 719-0154. *A clearinghouse for breast cancer information.*

16. EAT TO LIVE

Spinach is a good source of vitamin C

E very meal you eat can affect the quality—and length—of your life. Yet it's surprising how little you probably know about nutrition. Does orange juice really supply vitamin C? Are bran muffins healthy? Do you need to eat meat to get protein?

To make the right decisions about what to eat, you have to know more about *what* you're eating.

FOOD FACTS

Here are a few of the hundreds of facts about everyday foods and nutrition that may surprise you:

• It's estimated that most Americans get nearly twice the daily amount of protein we need. Studies show that the more protein people eat, the more calcium they excrete. This may explain why countries with the highest protein consumption—like ours—also have the highest rates of osteoporosis.

• The average American consumes 1/3 lb. of sugar *every day.* About 70% of it is "hidden" in processed foods. Check labels for sugars like: sucrose (table sugar, refined from sugarcane or beets), lactose (milk sugar), fructose (fruit sugar), dextrose, glucose, maltose and galactose.

• Drinking a glass of orange juice is less nutritious than eating an orange. Whole fruit contains fewer calories, and juice loses the fiber. Studies show that fiber helps to regulate metabolism of carbohydrates, so sugar in fruit is absorbed more slowly than the same sugar in fruit juice.

SIMPLE THINGS YOU CAN DO

1. Know What to Look For

• If you don't already know them, learn about nutrition basics. Get a book on nutrition from a library or bookstore (there are many to choose from), or contact the Resources below.

2. Protect Yourself

• Eat a balanced diet. According to the USDA, "You need more than 40 different nutrients for good health. These nutrients should come from a variety of foods, not from a few highly-fortified foods or supplements."

• A daily multiple vitamin and mineral supplement containing 100% of the RDA may be good for you if your diet is deficient in certain areas, but vitamin pills are no substitute for healthy eating.

• Remember that 55 to 60% of total calories consumed should come from carbohydrates, with emphasis on complex carbohydrates such as breads, pastas, cereals, potatoes, dried beans, peas and other legumes. In countries where heart disease is rare, 65-85% of the calories are carbohydrates.

• The recommended daily quota is 20 to 30 grams of fiber . A serving of some ultra-high-fiber cereals can supply 10 grams or more. Other good sources of fiber: fruit and vegetables, especially prunes and beans.

• Instead of making meat the center of your meals, try eating more vegetables and grains.

• Don't let words like "light" or "lite" fool you. The terms have no legal meaning, and are just as likely to refer to taste, texture, or appearance as they are to calorie or fat content.

RESOURCES

• **Center for Science in the Public Interest.** 1875 Connecticut Ave., Washington DC, 20009. *They offer numerous publications, including a newsletter called "Nutrition Action Health Letter," available for $19.95 a year. Write for information.*

• **Food and Drug Administration,** Consumer Inquiries. 5600 Fishers Lane Rockville, Maryland 20857. *Answers inquiries and supplies publications related to food and drug safety.*

• *The Tufts University Guide to Total Nutrition.* (Harper-Collins, 1991.)

17. CHECK YOUR CHOLESTEROL

According to a recent poll, more than 75% of Americans aren't sure what their cholesterol levels should be.

A lot of Americans are concerned about cholesterol—but don't know what it is.

According to the American Heart Association, "Cholesterol is a soft, fat-like substance found in all your body's cells. It's an important part of a healthy body because it's used to form cell membranes, certain hormones and other necessary tissues. The problem occurs when you have too much of it."

When there's too much cholesterol in your blood, it begins to build up on the artery walls, narrowing them and obstructing the flow of blood. This condition is known as "atherosclerosis." If the artery becomes totally blocked, you'll have a heart attack.

Most of us don't know whether we have too much cholesterol in our blood or not. But it's easy to find out. All it takes is a simple blood test.

CHOLESTEROL FACTS

• The cholesterol in your body comes from two main sources. Your liver manufactures some of it from fats, proteins, and carbohydrates. The rest is actually contained in animal products you eat. Vegetables don't contain cholesterol.

• Your liver manufactures enough cholesterol to meet all your body's needs. So you don't need the extra cholesterol contained in eggs, meat, and dairy products. Plus, the more saturated fat or hydrogenated oil you eat, the more cholesterol your liver produces.

• There are two main kinds of cholesterol traveling in your bloodstream: LDL (low-density lipoprotein) delivers cholesterol throughout your body to build cells. HDL (high-density lipoprotein) takes LDL cholesterol back to the liver for further processing or removal.

SIMPLE THINGS YOU CAN DO

1. Know What to Look For

• Blood cholesterol tests measure the total amount of cholesterol in your blood. A reading of less than 200 is considered low-risk.

• 200 to 239 is considered "borderline-high." The American Heart Association says "your chances of having a heart attack are nearly double those of someone whose level is well under 200." About 40% of American adults are in the group.

• If your level is 240 or over, your cholesterol level is definitely a problem. Your risk of having a heart attack is higher.

2. Get a Test

• Starting at age 20, check your cholesterol at least every 5 years.

• Get it checked by a doctor or other health-care professional; if it's not administered properly, the test may be inaccurate. For example, "finger-stick" tests offered at malls or supermarkets have been found to be inaccurate more than 50% of the time.

• Blood cholesterol can vary by as much as 20-40 points from one day to the next, so the best diagnosis is based on at least two tests taken on different days, a month or two apart.

• Discuss the results of your test with your doctor. If you have very high cholesterol, you'll probably need further tests to separate out the LDL and HDL levels. This information will help you determine how to lower it. Your doctor may recommend a change in eating habits, a weight loss program (see p. 82) , regular aerobic exercise (p. 24), more soluble fiber (p. 37), or quitting smoking (p. 86).

RESOURCES

• **The American Heart Association (AHA),** National Center, 7320 Greenville Ave., Dallas, TX 75231; (800) 527-6941. *Write or call for free pamphlet,* Cholesterol and Your Heart.

18. FINDING DR. RIGHT

In a UCLA School of Medicine survey, 85% of the people who responded had changed doctors in the past 5 years or were thinking of changing.

If you're feeling healthy, why not see a doctor?

That may sound strange, but if you don't have a regular doctor yet—or you're not happy with the one you do have—the best time to look is when you're feeling well, and there's time to consider all your alternatives.

SIMPLE THINGS YOU CAN DO

1. Plan Ahead

• Make a list of preferences. For example, does it matter if your doctor is male or female? Do you want someone older or someone just out of medical school who knows the latest technology?

• If you belong to an HMO, find out about their policy on selecting and switching doctors.

• Get referrals. Ask friends; a recommendation from a satisfied patient is one of the best tips you can get. A medical society or consumer affairs group can provide a list of doctors in your area.

2. Know What to Look For

• Call each referred doctor's office and get some basic information: Are they located near you? Can they be reached after office hours? How long does it take to get an appointment? Will they accept your insurance? Is the doctor affiliated with a hospital near you?

• Schedule a get-acquainted visit. It gives you a chance to find out if the doctor is a good listener and if you're comfortable with him or her. Your ability to confide in a doctor can make all the difference in getting the best possible health care.

RESOURCE

• How to Select the Right Doctor. *A 15-page brochure, free from Georgetown Medical Directory, 2233 Wisconsin Ave. NW, Suite 333, Washington, DC 20007.*

19. EAT FIBER

What has no nutrients and is basically undigestible...but is an important part of a healthy diet? Fiber—the "roughage" found in fruits, vegetables, grains and beans, that helps move food through the body. It's been credited with a long list of preventive health benefits, including lowering blood cholesterol levels, and reducing the risk of colon cancer. And because it lowers your blood cholesterol, it reduces the risk of heart attacks and strokes.

FIBER FACTS

There are two types of fiber:

• *Insoluble* fibers are found mainly in whole grains and the outside, or skin, of seeds, fruits, and beans. Studies show that these fibers may help prevent colorectal cancer. They absorb food like a sponge and move it through the bowel—decreasing the amount of cancer-causing substances that come in contact with the bowel wall.

• *Soluble* fibers are found in fruits, vegetables, seeds, brown rice, barley, and oats. They may lower cholesterol by adhering to fatty acids and reducing the amount of fat absorbed into the blood-stream.

SIMPLE THINGS YOU CAN DO

1. Know What to Look For

• Consult a nutrition book about sources and amounts of fiber, or call the American Cancer Society (800-ACS-2345). Ask for a copy of their free brochure: *Eating Smart*. It includes a list of foods and how much fiber they contain, as well as meal planning tips.

• Be sure your diet contains enough fiber; the FDA recommends a daily dose of 25-30 grams. Then *gradually* add more, if you need it.

• To be sure you get enough of both types of fiber, eat a wide variety of high-fiber foods.

• Caution: Just because a food is high in fiber doesn't mean it's good for you. Some high-fiber foods, like bran muffins, may also be high in fat (see p. 52)

20. WALK FOR EXERCISE

Walking is America's most popular form of excercise.

If you've been thinking about exercising, but just can't bear the thought of sweating in aerobics classes or working out in a gym, here's a simple alternative: Take a walk.

A brisk stroll down the street will help get your blood pumping, your heart beating, and your muscles working. It can make you feel better, fight disease, and, studies have shown, help you live longer.

SAVE YOUR LIFE

• Brisk walking is less wearing on your body than many other types of exercise, like jogging. "When people jog," explains one expert, "they land with 3 or 4 times their body weight....In walking, by definition, you always have one foot on the ground. You land with only one to one and a half times your weight."

• Mile for mile, walking burns the same number of calories as running. It also raises metabolic rates for 1 to 4 hours after exercising.

• According to Dr. James Rippe, a brisk 45-minute walk, four times a week, will burn off 18 lbs. of fat in a year if your diet doesn't change.

• Many studies indicate that walking lowers blood pressure and cholesterol levels, and helps control diabetes. "It doesn't really matter whether you walk slowly or fast," says one expert. "You still reduce your risk of coronary disease." One study showed that women who walked three miles a day, five days a week, reduced their risk of heart disease by as much as 18%.

• Walking improves your mental health, too. Researchers at the University of Massachusetts Center for Health and Fitness have found that at any pace, walking relieves anxiety.

SIMPLE THINGS YOU CAN DO

1. Know How to Walk

• Walking becomes aerobic exercise when you walk fast enough to bring your heartbeat up to its "target rate." (See p. 24.)

• Use the "talk test." If you're walking fast enough to be breathing hard, but not too fast to have a conversation comfortably, you're probably walking at a good, healthy pace. If you're too out of breath to carry on a conversation, you're walking too fast.

• Some experts recommend walking 20 minutes, four times a week, at a comfortable pace. "It takes about 20 minutes for your body to begin realizing the 'training effects' of sustained exercise," says one.

• Set a routine—walk at the same time each day.

• As your condition improves, increase time and pace.

• Remember: Your speed isn't as important as how long you walk.

• Don't be discouraged if you're out of shape. Experts say it takes only a month of conditioning to make up for each year of inactivity.

2. Plan Ahead

• Don't let the weather keep you from walking: Look for an indoor track or check local shopping malls. Many now have walking programs sponsored by the American Heart Association.

• Check with your local parks and recreation department. They may have a list of walking paths.

RESOURCES

• **The President's Council on Physical Fitness and Sports,** Superintendent of Documents, Government Printing Office, Washington, DC 20402-9325. *Write for their excellent brochure,* Walking for Exercise and Pleasure ($1.00).

• **The American Heart Association.** *Contact your local branch for free copies of the* Target Heart Rate Poster *and* Walking For A Healthy Heart.

• *The Walking Magazine,* Attn: Walking Club Coordinator, 9-11 Harcourt St., Boston, MA 02116. *For a free list of walking clubs in your area, send a SASE. The magazine is available at newstands.*

• *Dr. James M. Rippe's Complete Book of Fitness Walking,* by James M. Rippe and Ann Ward. (Prentice Hall Press, 1989).

• *Walking Medicine,* by Gary Yanker and Kathy Burton. (McGraw-Hill, 1990).

21. LEARN ABOUT AIDS

*An estimated 70% of HIV-infected people
worldwide got it from heterosexual activity.*

How much do you know about AIDS? Do you know, for example, how it's spread and why it's so deadly? Do you know how you can prevent it...and who's at risk?

AIDS is not "someone else's" disease. Anyone can get it, and everyone needs to know about it.

WHAT DO YOU KNOW?

Here are a few simple questions about AIDS. If you can't answer them, you may not know how to protect yourself from this deadly disease.

True or False?

1. Anyone who's infected with the virus that causes AIDS sees some symptoms right away.

Answer: No. The incubation period for the *human immunodeficiency virus* (HIV) is 7-11 years; anyone who hasn't been tested can have it and not know it yet. (The virus usually shows up in tests after 3-6 months.) In fact, the Centers for Disease Control estimate that of the 1.5 million Americans thought to be infected with HIV, about 75% may not know it.

2. You can catch AIDS from shaking hands with someone.

Answer: No, there's not enough HIV in sweat to be contagious.

3. You can get AIDS through all kinds of close sexual contact.

Answer: True, AIDS is spread through sexual contact—the HIV is in blood, semen, and vaginal fluids. Anal sex is particularly high-risk, because it tends to tear membranes.

4. Mosquitoes transmit AIDS.

Answer: False.

5. If someone with AIDS handles your food, you can catch it.

Answer: Polls show that 25% of Americans fear they can get AIDS from a cook, but experts say it's a myth. It's not passed on in food, even if an HIV-infected chef suffers a cut while preparing it.

6. Sharing a needle to inject drugs can give you HIV.

Answer: True, if shared wth infected person(s).

7. You can avoid getting AIDS by using a condom.

Answer: They're not foolproof, but they usually work. However, it's important to use latex—not animal skin—condoms. Animal skin condoms have tiny pores through which HIV can pass. To make condoms more effective, use a water-based lubricant, like K-Y Jelly (never oil-based lubricants, which dissolve latex), and a spermicide, like nonoxynol-9. Spermicides kill HIV in lab tests. Note: Other birth control devices, like cervical caps and IUDs, offer *no* protection from HIV.

SIMPLE THINGS YOU CAN DO

1. Know Your Risk

• Learn about AIDS. Contact the resources below, or check your library.

2. Protect yourself.

• Practice safer sex—use a condom. Don't share needles or other drug paraphernalia. Avoid exposure to blood of infected persons.

• If you think you're at risk for HIV infection, talk to your doctor, or call an AIDS hotline. They'll tell you where to get a confidential (or even anonymous) HIV blood test.

• Even if you find you are HIV positive, there are many things you can do to keep yourself as healthy as possible—from getting regular checkups to dietary changes, from simple vaccinations (such as flu) to AZT and other drugs that may slow the onset of AIDS.

3. Volunteer With a Local AIDS Service Group (See P. 66.)

RESOURCES

• **National AIDS Information Hotline.** *Has three toll-free numbers: (800) 342-AIDS for people who speak English, (800) 344-SIDA for those who speak Spanish, and (800) AIDS-TTY, a TTY/TTD hotline for the hearing impaired.*

• **U.S. Public Health Service, Centers for Disease Control,** P.O. Box 6003, Rockville, MD 20850. *Send for a free copy of "Understanding AIDS: A Message from the Surgeon General."*

22. LEARN THE SIGNS OF A HEART ATTACK

About 4,000 Americans suffer heart attacks every day—1 every 20 seconds.

Michael Brunsfeld was 40 years old when he had a heart attack. He had no personal history of heart problems—and no heart attacks in his family.

"Three days before it happened," he says, "I felt a strange sensation in my arm. I certainly didn't associate it with anything relating to my heart, but I didn't know *what* it was. I'd just had the flu, so I thought it was a weird flu symptom.

"For three successive days I had these symptoms. Finally, I called the emergency room at a local hospital. They said it sounded like heart problems and suggested that if it happened again, I should go to the emergency room right away.

"I went to the emergency room the next day and while I was there, I started to feel the worst symptoms of all. I found out that I was having a heart attack...while I was in the emergency room."

Michael was lucky; if he hadn't been at the hospital, he might have died. But he'd also had three days' warning, and didn't know it. If you had symptoms of a heart attack, would you recognize them? It could make all the difference.

SAVE YOUR LIFE

• Most heart attacks occur between 7 and 10 a.m.

• About 5% of all heart attacks occur in people under age 40, and 45% occur in people under 65.

• An American male has a one-in-five chance of having a heart attack before the age of 65.

• Many people who experience the symptoms of a heart attack will deny the signs and try to rationalize that it's something minor, like indigestion. Most deaths associated with heart attacks occur within two hours of the first pain, so getting immediate attention is the key to survival and recovery.

SIMPLE THINGS YOU CAN DO

1. Know What to Look For

• According to the American Heart Association, the symptoms of a heart attack vary, but these are the most common ones:

√ Intense pain, or a feeling of pressure or tightness, in the center of the chest that lasts for two minutes or more

√ Pain spreading to the shoulders, neck, jaw, arms, back or upper abdomen.

√ Sometimes these are accompanied by lightheadedness, fainting, sweating, nausea, and/or shortness of breath.

Note: Short stabbing pains that last for less than 10 seconds are *usually* not a sign of a heart attack.

2. Get Help, If You Need It

• In a heart attack emergency, call 911, or an emergency medical service. In your area that could be either the fire department or an ambulance service. *The goal is to get to a hospital emergency room as quickly as possible.*

• It's better to call an ambulance than to be driven by a friend or family member. Ambulance drivers are less likely to have an accident on the way to the hospital, and they carry equipment so they can respond to an emergency while on route.

3. Plan Ahead

• Do a little investigating before an emergency strikes. Find out which hospitals are nearest your home and office, and keep 24-hour, emergency cardiac care phone numbers near all your phones. The AHA offers phone stickers for this purpose.

• If you don't know CPR, consider taking a class. There's a chance you could use it to save a heart attack victim's life by keeping their heart beating until the ambulance arrives. (See p. 78 for information on CPR.)

RESOURCE

• **The American Heart Association (AHA),** National Center, 7320 Greenville Ave., Dallas, TX 75231; (800) 527-6941 *or local chapters. Offers numerous brochures on heart health. The first five brochures are free, and then a nominal fee is charged.*

23. INSTALL SMOKE DETECTORS

*In one year, 90% of all fire fatalities occurred
in homes without smoke detectors.*

B elieve it or not, fire strikes a home somewhere in the U.S.
every 47 seconds. That's why it's so important to install
smoke detectors in *your* home.

SAVE YOUR LIFE

• Fire is the second leading cause of death in U.S. homes.

• According to the National Fire Protection Association, installing smoke detectors cuts the risk of dying in a home fire by 50%.

• Unfortunately, experts estimate that one-third of the smoke detectors in U.S. homes are not in working order.

SIMPLE THINGS YOU CAN DO

Install Smoke Alarms

• Experts recommend putting one outside each bedroom and on each additional level of the house—including the basement and attic. If you sleep with the bedroom door closed, or if you smoke, it's a good idea to install one in your bedroom.

• Don't put smoke detectors within 3 feet of a vent or window, because drafts can keep smoke from reaching them. Don't put them in bathrooms, because water vapor also prevents smoke from reaching them. Also: Don't put them in corners.

• Test smoke detectors every 6 months to make sure they're working. Set aside a special day—such as daylight savings time— to do the test. Replace batteries and clean the unit at least once a year.

• Vacuum the grillwork of your smoke detector frequently, so smoke particles can enter.

RESOURCES

"Smoke Detectors—A Fire Safety Basic." National Fire Protection Association Public Affairs Office, Dept. TFH, PO Box 9101, ·
1 Batterymarch Park, Quincy, MA 02269; (800) 344-3555.

WITH A LITTLE

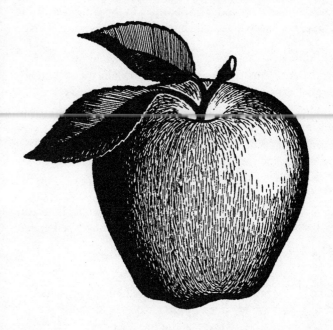

EFFORT

24. SAVE YOUR SKIN

One in six Americans will develop some form of skin cancer.

T here's nothing like going to the beach or a swimming pool and lying out in the sun. But now, "soaking up some rays," even in everyday activities, could be costly. Skin cancer has become the most common form of cancer in the U.S. today...and nine times out of ten it's caused by too much exposure to the sun.

SAVE YOUR LIFE

• More cases of skin cancer are reported annually than all other cancers combined. Over 600,000 people will get it this year.

• All skin cancers are treatable and most are curable when brought to the attention of a doctor in their early stages.

• If even the most dangerous form of skin cancer is found and removed early enough, there's about a 90% survival rate. Despite this, 8,500 people die from skin cancer each year.

• Self-exams can aid early detection. According to one report, about 70% of the time a dangerous skin cancer is found in its early stages, it's because a patient has identified it through a self-exam.

THE SUN AND CANCER

• Skin cancer is caused by the sun's ultraviolet (UV) light. Every exposure to UV rays is "stored" in the skin. Unlike tans, which eventually fade, damage done by UV exposure is cumulative.

• There are two kinds of UV light—UVA and UVB. Ultraviolet B is the shorter-wave light that causes immediate sunburns...and eventually skin cancer. UVA, which also comes from the sun (and is used in tanning salons), penetrates more deeply. It damages blood vessels and enhances the cancer-causing potential of UVB.

• In the 1930s, only one in 1,500 people developed the most deadly form of skin cancer. Today, the figure is 1 in 105. Experts blame this increase to the tanning craze that began in the 1950s. The gradual destruction of the Earth's ozone layer may also be a factor.

• Children are particularly at risk. By the time they're 18, most will have received 50-80% of their lifetime sun exposure.

SIMPLE THINGS YOU CAN DO

1. Know Your Risk

• If you sunburn easily and have a hard time getting tan, you're especially vulnerable to skin cancer. If you have fair skin, red or blonde hair, and light-colored eyes, you are at higher risk.

• If you got a severe, blistering sunburn during childhood, you're more likely to get the most deadly form of skin cancer later in life.

• If a member of your immediate family had skin cancer, you're at risk. About 10% of skin cancer cases run in families.

2. Know What to Look For

• 80% of all skin cancers occur on the face, head and neck.

• Check regularly for signs of skin cancer. Every month, examine spots, moles, and blemishes on your body.

• If you notice a change, or anything unusual (for example, a mole wider than a 1/4-inch pencil eraser that grows in diameter, is different shades of color, or has rough and uneven borders), see your doctor or dermatologist immediately.

3. Protect Yourself

• Cut back on how much sun you get. Be most careful between 10 a.m. and 3 p.m., when the sun's UV rays are most intense.

• Wear a hat to protect your face and head (especially if you're bald). If possible, cover your arms and legs. Be careful on overcast days; as much as 85% of the sun's ultraviolet rays can penetrate clouds.

• Use sunscreen, even if you're not on the beach. Apply it 30-45 minutes before exposure. Experts recommend a Sun Protection Factor (SPF) of at least 15. A higher rating isn't necessary, as long as you apply sunscreen liberally. An average adult should use about an ounce per application. Apply evenly to all exposed skin.

• Note: Sunscreens are formulated today to protect against UVB. But sunscreens rated SPF 15 or higher contain ingredients that provide some protection against UVA.

RESOURCES

• Skin Cancer Foundation, Box 561, Dept. AB, New York, NY 10156. *Send a self-addressed, stamped envelope for free brochures.*

25. DRINKING & DRIVING

In the time it takes you to read this sentence, there will be an alcohol- or drug-related traffic accident in the United States.

According to the National Safety Council, driving under the influence of alcohol is "the most common violent crime in the U.S." There are 2 million alcohol-related car accidents every year, and about 22,000 people are killed in them.

You may not think this applies to you, if you never drive when you're "drunk." But according to experts, even as little as .05% blood alcohol content—half the legal limit—can cause "significant interruption of brain and body functions." This means that even if you've only had a drink or two, you could be driving impaired—putting yourself and others in danger—without realizing it.

ONE FOR THE ROAD?

• Statistically, you have a 40% chance of being involved in an alcohol-related crash.

• About 24% of all drivers involved in fatal crashes are "driving-impaired."

• On an average weekend night, one in ten drivers is "under the influence."

• Drunk driving is a leading cause of death for Americans ages 16-24. Young drivers account for more than a third of all alcohol-related crashes.

• It's a myth that coffee, fresh air, a cold shower, or any other "remedy" will sober you up. The only way to get sober is to give your body time to get rid of the alcohol—about an hour for each drink if you weigh over 150 pounds. If you weigh less, it could take longer.

SIMPLE THINGS YOU CAN DO

1. If You Drink, Don't Drive

• It's still the best solution. There's really no way you can tell if you've had too much.

• Wait, call a taxi, ask a friend for a ride, or spend the night where you are.

2. Protect Your Friends

• If you think a friend is drunk, insist on driving him or her home, calling a taxi for them, or having them spend the night.

• If you're giving a party, remember these tips:

√ Don't force drinks on guests. They may accept drinks just to please you. And pace the serving, so they won't drink too fast.

√ Serve high-protein snacks (see below).

√ Offer non-alcoholic drinks. Near the end of the party, serve *only* non-alcoholic drinks, so people will have a chance to metabolize the alcohol they've already drunk.

3. Protect Your Children

• If you have teenage drivers at home, make sure they understand that safety is more important to you than getting home on time. Tell them that it's never okay to drink and drive.

• Offer to drive them home whenever they need it, and give them a number where you can be reached, or give them cab fare.

4. Plan Ahead

• If you're in a situation where you'll be drinking, take it slowly. Pass up rounds or switch to non-alcoholic drinks. Be prepared to call a cab or ask a friend to drive you home. If nobody can drive you home, wait awhile before you drive.

• Eat when you drink. Food can slow the absorption of alcohol into the bloodstream, but only if you eat it before or while you're drinking. After a certain point, it won't stop you from getting drunk. High-protein foods (cheese, meat) are best because they take longer to digest.

• If you're drinking with friends, assign a *designated driver* who agrees not to drink and will drive everyone else home. In Europe, designated drivers put car keys in an empty glass in front of them so people won't offer them drinks.

RESOURCES

• Mothers Against Drunk Driving (MADD), 511 E. John Carpenter Fwy., Suite 700, Irving, TX 75062-8187. *Write for free information.*

• Students Against Driving Drunk, P.O. Box 800, Marlboro, MA 01752; (508) 481-3568. *Free information for young people.*

26. BON VOYAGE

*It's estimated that a third of all travelers get some
sort of illness while they're away from home.*

E very year, more than 30 million Americans travel abroad. If
you're planning to visit another country, it's as important to
take certain health-related precautions as it is to make hotel
reservations or get traveler's checks. Potentially fatal diseases that
are rare in the U.S., like cholera, yellow fever, and typhoid, may be
common abroad.

THE FACTS ABROAD

• The Centers for Disease Control (CDC) report that in 1991,
Americans contracted typhoid and cholera while traveling. Both
illnesses could have been avoided with proper vaccinations.

• Malaria is a health risk in some tropical countries. More than
80% of U.S. cases originate in sub-Saharan Africa.

• As in the U.S., the major threat of getting AIDS when traveling
is through sexual activity with an infected person. But AIDS can
also be acquired through contact with local medical systems. In
some developing countries, needles may be reused, and blood or
blood products may not be properly screened.

SIMPLE THINGS YOU CAN DO

1. Know Your Risk

• Get up-to-date immunization advice from the CDC International Travelers Hotline at (404) 332-4559 (rather than your local doctor). Or make an appointment at a special travel clinic. Some
countries require proof of immunization.

• For information on preventing diseases for which there is no
immunization, call the CDC Hotline at (404) 332-4555. To speak
with a CDC malaria specialist, call (404) 488-4046.

• Consult the CDC's *Health Information for International Travel* or
Fielding's Traveler's Medical Companion (see Resources) for information on eating and drinking abroad. Diseases like cholera, hepatitis,
and typhoid are transmitted by contaminated food and water.

2. Protect Yourself

• Get immunized. Some vaccines require a series of shots; others need time to become active. Travel experts suggest starting immunizations at least 6-8 weeks before departure date.

3. Plan Ahead

• Pack a sufficient supply of any medicine you take regularly. Put it in a carry-on bag that you'll keep with you, so it won't get lost or delayed.

• To avoid having medicine confiscated by customs agents, keep it in original containers. Bring a doctor's note stating the need for it.

• Carry phone numbers of your pharmacist and doctor, in case you lose medications. Another good idea: Take along written prescriptions, in case your supply of medicine is lost or damaged.

• Keep a copy of your itinerary for at least a year so you can show it to your doctor if you get sick. It's not uncommon to become ill after you return home. Some diseases, like malaria, may not cause symptoms for as long as 6-12 months.

RESOURCES

• *Health Information for International Travel—an up-to-date guide about health risks abroad—is available for $5 by writing the CDC, Superintendent of Documents, Washington, DC 20402. Also offered: International Travelers Hotline, (404) 332-4559.*

• **International Association for Medical Assistance to Travelers,** 417 Center St., Lewiston, NY 14092. *Publishes a worldwide directory of English-speaking physicians trained in Canada or the U.S. Also offers free leaflets. Donations appreciated.*

• *Fielding's Traveler's Medical Companion,* by Eden Graber and Paula M. Siegel (Fielding / Morrow, 1990).

• *The Pocket Doctor: Your Ticket to Good Health While Traveling,* by Stephen Bezruchka, M.D. (Mountaineers Books, 1988). *Available by calling (800) 553-4453 or writing 1011 S.W. Klickitat Way, Suite 107, Seattle, WA 98134; also available in stores.*

• **The Traveler's Health and Immunization Services,** 148 Highland Ave., Newton, MA 02160. *For a free directory of travel health clinics near you, send a stamped, self-addressed, 8-1/2" x 11" envelope.*

27. TRIM THE FAT

According to one expert, if U.S. women ate half as much fat as they currently do, "breast cancer alone coould decline by as much as 60%."

I f you're a typical American, you get around 40% of your calories from fat. Most of it is unnecessary—and worse, it's linked to serious health problems like heart disease and cancer.

The solution is to cut down. The FDA recommends that no more than 30% of your daily calories come from fat. Other sources suggest as little as 20% or 25%.

Once you've made up your mind to make a change, it's going to take some research to figure out where the fat is…because 50%-65% of the fat in a normal American diet is "hidden" in cheese, fried foods, etc. The challenge is to find the fat in *your* diet…and trim it.

FAT FACTS

There are three kinds of fat:

• *Saturated* fat is clearly linked to hardening of the arteries, excessive cholesterol, heart disease and strokes. It's contained in meat and dairy products, palm oil, coconut oil, cocoa butter and any oil that has been "hydrogenated."

• *Polyunsaturated fat*, found in corn, safflower, soybean and sunflower oils. For a long time, nutritionists recommended polyunsaturated fat because it appeared to reduce cholesterol levels, but new studies show it may neutralize "good" cholesterol in the body as well as bad (see p. 34), and some studies have implicated it in the development of breast, ovarian and prostate tumors.

• *Monounsaturated* fat is found in olive, peanut, sesame, walnut and canola oils. Of all the fats, this seems to be the least likely to cause heart and cancer problems.

• All fats are equally fattening; each contains 9 calories per gram. By contrast, protein and carbohydrates each have 4 calories a gram.

SIMPLE THINGS YOU CAN DO

1. Know What to Look For

To find out how much fat is in the food you eat:

- Use a guide that lists fat content of a wide variety of foods, like *The American Heart Association Fat and Cholesterol Counter* (published by Random House, $3.50).
- Learn to read labels for fat content:

√ Bring your calculator to the market.

√ Pick up a package. Look at the nutritional information.

√ Find the listing for "Fat per serving." It's always expressed in grams.

√ Multiply that number by 9 (the number of calories per gram of fat). That gives you the total number of calories per serving that are from fat.

√ Divide that number by the number of total calories per serving (also listed on the package). For example, if there are 54 total calories per serving in a box of crackers, and 27 calories of fat (3 grams), then you divide 27 by 54. The number you'll get is .50...or 50%. That's the percentage of calories in your crackers that come from fat.

2. Look for Alternatives

- Once you know where the fat in your diet is, find a way to replace it. For example:

√ Even "2% lowfat milk" actually gets 35% of its calories from fat because nutrients are listed by percentage of weight—not by calories. Alternative: Drink skim milk.

√ Canned tuna packed in water has 2/3 less fat than tuna in oil.

√ Eat vegetables raw or steamed, instead of frying them.

√ Trimming skin from light-meat chicken—before or after cooking—cuts total fat content by over 50%.

√ Use less butter—a teaspoon instead of a tablespoon, for instance.

RESOURCE

- Information on an extensive variety of foods is available in "Nutritive Value of Foods" from the USDA. *For a copy, send $3.75 to Superintendent of Documents, U.S. Government Printing Office, Washington, D.C. 20402-9325. Ask for "Home and Garden Bulletin Number 72."*

28. STOP STROKES

The U.S. population averages one stroke a minute and a death from stroke every three minutes.

You probably know that strokes are a major health risk for American adults. But did you know that many strokes are actually preventable...and if a stroke does occur, you may get warning signals in advance? Unfortunately, studies show that only 8% of people who get strokes can recognize these symptoms...so most don't seek medical attention until an average of *13 hours* after the symptoms appear. That may be too late.

WHAT IS A STROKE?

• A stroke is a disruption of blood flow to the brain. Without a source of fresh blood, brain cells are deprived of oxygen and rapidly die. Once dead, these cells are gone for good; and it only takes 4-5 minutes for irreversible damage to occur.

• Strokes can be classified in two ways. One type of stroke occurs when a vessel ruptures and causes bleeding in the brain; the other occurs when a clot obstructs a blood vessel and keeps blood from reaching the brain. The outcome of a stroke depends on which section of the brain has been damaged.

• Strokes are the largest cause of adult disability and the third leading cause of death in the U.S.

SIMPLE THINGS YOU CAN DO

1. Know Your Risk

• According to the National Stroke Association, 40-70% of people who suffer strokes have a history of high blood pressure.

• Men are more likely than women to have a stroke.

• Smokers are 2-3 times more likely to have a stroke than non-smokers. Smokers with high blood pressure are *20 times* more likely to suffer a stroke.

• If someone in your family has had a stroke, you're at a higher risk.

• African-Americans get strokes more often than Caucasians.

• A stroke is more likely to occur as you get older, and the risk doubles each decade after age 55. Two-thirds of all strokes occur in people over age 65.

• According to a report from the Framingham Heart Study, people who are even 10% over their ideal body weight are at an increased risk for stroke.

2. Know What to Look For

• Four out of five stroke victims suffer a *transient ischemic attack* (TIA), or a "mini-stroke," just before having a serious, debilitative stroke. TIAs can be mild, and usually pass quickly, but don't ignore them. If you experience any of the following symptoms, see a doctor right away, especially if you're in a high-risk group.

 √ Numbness or weakness in your face, arm, hand, or leg

 √ Temporary blindness, or blurred vision in one or both eyes

 √ Difficulty speaking, understanding speech, or swallowing

 √ Dizziness, fainting, or loss of balance

 √ Sudden, unexplained headaches

• The greatest risk is in the first week after a TIA occurs, but if you think you may have had a TIA a while ago, it's still important to get medical attention—several studies indicate that people can go up to five years after having a TIA before having a major stroke.

3. Protect Yourself

• The same things that reduce your risk of having a heart attack can keep you from having a stroke. Watch your blood pressure (see p. 14), cut cholesterol (p. 34) and saturated fats. (p. 52), quit smoking (P. 86), drink alcohol moderately (p. 88), exercise regularly (p. 24), and watch your weight (p. 82) .

RESOURCES

• **National Stroke Association**, 300 East Hampden Ave., Suite 240, Englewood, CO 80110-2654, (303) 762-9922; *Numerous services and free pamphlets available, including support for stroke victims.*

• **The American Heart Association.** *Contact your local branch for several brochures on stroke including "Facts About Strokes" and "Recovering" from a Stroke. Cost is $.25-$1.00 for each.*

29. DANGER: POISON

More than 250,000 everyday household products are potentially poisonous.

I n the comics, you can always tell when something is poison—
it comes in a black bottle, and it's labeled with a skull and
crossbones. But in real life, poisons aren't so easy to spot. Even
things we use every day—cleansers, medicine, cosmetics, etc.—can
be lethal under certain circumstances...especially for children.

About 1.7 million poisonings are reported each year; one million
of these involve children under 6 years old. The majority of
accidental poisonings—about 91% of them—occur at home. Fortunately, 80% of them can be successfully treated at home, too.

Taking a few basic precautions with household products, and
knowing what to do in a poison emergency, could save a life.

SIMPLE THINGS YOU CAN DO

1. Know Your Risk

• Accidental poisonings involving adults happen most often when
poison is stored in a drinking container, like a soda bottle or glass.
All it takes is a sip; one teaspoon of antifreeze can kill an adult.

• If your child ingests anything that is "non-food," they're at risk.
Call the poison control center.

• Ingestion isn't the only danger. Children may put their hands in
chemicals which can burn the skin—or their eyes, if they rub them.

2. Know What to Look For

• Contact your local poison control center or write to the
Pittsburgh Poison Center (see Resources) for a list of commonly
used household products that can be potential poisons.

3. Poison-Proof Your Home

• Keep drugs, chemicals, pesticides, and cleaners in original containers. Make sure they're properly labeled. If an original container
leaks, put the whole thing in a larger container and re-label it.

• A number of common plants—such as hyacinth, azalea, and
wisteria—are extremely poisonous. Kids (and pets) sometimes eat
the leaves. Call a local poison center for info about your plants. If

any are poisonous, keep them out of children's reach.

• Use safety latches on cabinets and drawers. Store hazardous products out of children's reach. This goes for toxics kept in the garage or basement as well—such as paint or bug sprays.

3. Protect Your Children

• Teach children which products can hurt them; put a "Mr. Yuk" sticker (see Resources) on all potentially harmful products.

• If you're interrupted while using anything potentially poisonous, take it with you. Accidents involving children often occur while an adult has a harmful product out of storage ...and is using it. For example, imagine you're polishing a dining room table, and the phone rings. While you answer it, your child could grab the polish.

• Use unscented cleaning products your child won't associate with food or beverages. Accidental poisonings often happen around mealtimes when kids are hungry and thirsty. Many household products (e.g., strawberry-scented kerosene oil) are colorful and smell good. Hungry children may think they're food and help themselves.

• Keep a bottle of syrup of ipecac (available at pharmacies) on hand to induce vomiting in case of poisoning. Use it *only* if instructed to do so by a poison center or physician; some poisons become *more* dangerous if vomiting occurs.

4. Plan Ahead

• Keep the number of your local poison center by the phone. In case of poisoning, the staff will tell you if hospital treatment is needed.

• If the poisoning can be safely treated at home, the poison center staff will tell you, step by step, exactly how to do it.

• If necessary, the poison center will refer you to the nearest hospital. They'll call ahead and provide the hospital with information about the patient and poison.

RESOURCES

• **Pittsburgh Poison Center**, Children's Hospital of Pittsburgh, 1 Children's Place, 3705 5th Ave., Pittsburgh, PA 15213. *One of America's leading poison control centers. Excellent materials on preventing accidental poisonings, including "Mr. Yuk" stickers. Send for free catalog.*

30. WEAR A BICYCLE HELMET

*In 1990, 580,000 bicyclists were treated for injuries in hospital
emergency rooms—an average of one serious injury per minute.*

Bicycling has become one of the most popular activities in the
U.S. It's estimated that 25 million adults and 20 million
children ride bikes at least once a week.

If you're like many people, you probably love your bike, but hate
wearing a helmet because it "looks funny" and is inconvenient to
put on. That's understandable…until you learn about how it can
save your life.

SAVE YOUR LIFE

• A good bicycle helmet protects you in three ways: It absorbs the
shock of a crash, distributes the force of the impact over the surface
of the helmet instead of the head, and protects the head from sharp
objects.

• In one year, about 125,000 cyclists—many of them children—
suffer head injuries. Most of these could be prevented by wearing
protective helmets.

• About 850 bicyclists die each year in accidents—90% of them in
collisions with motor vehicles. Head injuries account for 75% of
these fatalities.

• According to a recent study in the *New England Journal of
Medicine,* bicycle helmets reduce the risk of head injuries by 85%.
They help reduce fatalities by more than 50%. Yet only 5-10% of
American bike riders regularly wear helmets.

SIMPLE THINGS YOU CAN DO

1. Know Your Risk

• Even low-speed crashes—5 mph or less—can result in permanent
brain damage if you're not wearing a helmet.

• "Head injuries generally occur not because of the speed," one
expert explains, "but because of vertical distance—how far your

head travels to hit the pavement. The average height of a person sitting on a bike is 5 feet. A fall from that distance can cause irreversible injury to the brain."

• If you fall, your head could hit the pavement in half a second. Blink once. That's about how long you'd have to protect your head if you weren't wearing a helmet.

2. Know What to Look For

• Get a helmet with a hard, smooth outer shell: it helps absorb and distribute the impact of an accident, reduces the chances of fracturing your skull, helps protect your head if you slide along pavement, and shields you from sharp objects.

• Helmets with soft outer shells tend to "stick" to pavement according to tests, increasing the risk of neck injury.

• Look for a helmet that's approved by the American National Standards Institute or Snell Memorial Foundation. These groups have reliable safety standards.

3. Protect Yourself

• If you crash, replace your helmet. Most helmets are designed to withstand the shock of an impact only once. Even if they look okay, they may not be structurally sound any more.

• Some manufacturers will replace a damaged helmet free if you send it to them for inspection.

4. Protect Your Children

• Teach them to wear helmets. Start the habit young with a child's first bicycle. Quality kids' helmets are only about $25.

• Let your child pick out the helmet. Kids are much more likely to wear a helmet they like.

• Give a helmet as a gift. Two million children receive bicycles as gifts each year in the U.S., but only 5% are also given helmets.

RESOURCES

• Bicycle Helmet Safety Institute, 4611 7th St. South, Arlington, VA 22204; (703) 486-0100. *Send $1 and a self-addressed, stamped envelope for a copy of "A Consumer's Guide to Bicycle Helmets."*

31. KNOW YOUR RISK FOR HEART DISEASE

Every year, more Americans die of heart disease than were killed in World Wars I and II, the Korean War, and Vietnam combined.

You've probably heard it before: Heart disease is the number-one killer in the U.S.

The best thing you can do to protect yourself is to learn the risks, and the simple lifestyle changes that can make a big difference.

HEART FACTS

• Your heart is probably smaller than you think—roughly the size of your clenched fist. But in the one minute it takes to read this page, it will pump 5 quarts of blood through your body.

• When your heart "beats," you're actually feeling it expanding to draw blood from the rest of the body, and then contracting to force it out again. Heart disease is any condition that affects your heart's ability to pump blood this way.

• The main cause of heart disease is *atherosclerosis*. Arteries become narrowed due to a buildup of fatty plaques (mostly cholesterol) on the inside of artery walls. This limits blood flow to one or more of the coronary arteries and can result in a heart attack.

• More than 5 million Americans have been diagnosed with heart disease. As many as 12 million more may be unaware they have it.

• Before age 60, one in five men and one in seventeen women will experience heart or coronary disease symptoms.

SIMPLE THINGS YOU CAN DO

1. Know Your Risk

• If heart disease runs in your family, you're 2-5 times more likely than average to have it too.

• Smoking increases your chance of heart attack by 2-4 times.

• Birth control pills may cause side effects related to increased cardiac risks, especially if you smoke.

• High blood pressure (see p. 14), high cholesterol (see p. 34), or diabetes increases your chances of heart disease.

• You're at risk if you're overweight. For example: One study found that women averaging just 10% higher than recommended weight levels face a 30% higher chance of a heart attack than women slightly below those levels. At 15-29% overweight, the risk is 80% higher; at 30% or more overweight, it's 230% higher.

2. Get a Test

• Check for "silent heart disease." Don't wait until you experience symptoms. If you're at high risk, doctors can use advanced medical testing (like treadmill stress tests) to detect it.

3. Protect Yourself

• Exercise regularly. Researchers at the Centers for Disease Control say "the nation's most common cardiac threat is physical inactivity." Studies suggest that burning an average of 200-300 calories a day in any form of recreation is the minimum needed to begin reducing your chance of a coronary. For maximum improvement, burn 2,000 calories a week. See Stay Active (p. 20), Walk for Exercise (p. 38), and Aerobic Exercise (p. 24).

• Eat right. The AHA recommends a "heart healthy" diet for all healthy people more than 2 years of age. See Resources for more information. Also see Trim The Fat (p. 52) and Eat to Live (p. 32).

• Take aspirin if your doctor approves it. There's evidence that daily use of aspirin can prevent heart attacks. The best dosage: 30 milligrams—less than half a dose of baby aspirin. *Remember:* aspirin is a drug and could possibly cause complications, so talk to your doctor before taking it.

RESOURCES

• **The American Heart Association (AHA),** National Center, 7320 Greenville Ave., Dallas, TX 75231; (800) 527-6941 *or local chapters. Offers numerous brochures on heart health. The first five brochures are free, and then a nominal fee is charged.*

• **National Heart, Lung and Blood Institute Information Center,** 7200 Wisconsin Ave., Box 329, Bethesda, MD 20814; (301) 951-3260. *Offers free brochures on heart disease risk and prevention.*

32. DRIVE DEFENSIVELY

Traffic accidents are the #1 killer of Americans ages one to forty-four.

How important is defensive driving? Consider who you're sharing the road with: In a 1991 survey, one-third of all drivers polled said that a flashing red traffic signal means "proceed with caution." It actually means "stop." One-fifth of them said it was "correct and safe" to back up on a freeway to make another attempt at a missed exit ramp. It's not. And another survey found that 3% of all drivers say they drive after drinking "all the time."

Every year about 50,000 people are killed and 3.4 million more are injured in automobile accidents. Studies show that up to 85% of these accidents could have been avoided. Your best protection is defensive driving—being ready for anything.

SIMPLE THINGS YOU CAN DO

1. Use the "Two-Second" Rule

• If you're driving on a street and the car in front of you has to come to a quick stop, it normally takes at least two seconds for you to react and stop your own car. The two-second rule builds a safe following distance between you and vehicles ahead. Here's how it works:

√ When the car in front of you passes a fixed object like a tree or telephone pole, start counting—*one thousand one, one thousand two*.

√ If your car reaches the fixed object before you finish counting, you're following too closely. Widen the gap.

√ If you're driving at highway speeds of 55 mph or more, you need more time to react. Give yourself three to four seconds.

√ If driving conditions are less than ideal—for example, if the road is wet or visibility is poor—allow at least four seconds of following distance.

2. Plan Ahead

• Be on the lookout for potential problems. Keep your eyes moving and look as far ahead as you can. Ask yourself, "What if?" What if that car suddenly pulls out? What if that child runs out in the street? What if traffic ahead comes to a stop? What if that car changes lanes without seeing you?

• Check behind you. Regularly scan your side and rearview mirrors (about every 6-8 seconds, according to AAA) to keep track of the traffic behind you. If you need to make a sudden lane change, you'll know if the lane is open.

• Be especially careful at intersections. About 40% of all urban accidents happen there. The National Safety Council's advice: approach intersections with your foot off the accelerator and over the brake pedal. Look left, then right, then left again before proceeding through; keep scanning until you're safely past the point of danger.

• "Behind the wheel, your mind should be on driving," says Rhett Price, Public Affairs Officer for the California Highway Patrol. "Driving takes total concentration. If you're distracted—for example, if your children are acting up, a bee gets inside your car—it's best to pull off the road."

RESOURCES

• "Defensive Driving: Managing Time and Space." Traffic Safety Department, American Automobile Assn., Falls Church, VA 22047. *Free with self-addressed, stamped envelope.*

• "How To Drive After Dark." National Safety Council, Dept. PR-P, 444 N. Michigan Ave., Chicago, IL 60611. *Send an SASE and ask for the brochure by name.*

• "Driving tips for older adults." American Optometric Association, Communications Center-P, 243 N. Lindbergh Blvd., St. Louis, MO 63141. *Send an SASE.*

• *55 Alive/Mature Driving. Sponsored by AARP. An 8-hour refresher driving course offered to people over the age of 50. Available in all 50 states. Cost: $8. If interested in taking the course, send a letter with name, address, county and phone number to AARP National Headquarters: 601 E Street, NW, Washington D.C., 20049. A local instructor will then contact you.*

33. GET A GOOD NIGHT'S SLEEP

It's estimated that 30-50 milion Americans suffer fom sleep disorders.

A re you getting enough sleep? According to recent polls, as many as a third of all Americans have sleeping problems that keep them up at night and drowsy during the day. Lack of sleep is always inconvenient...but it can also cause physical problems. A prolonged lack of sleep can make you prone to illness...or accidents. And the less you sleep, the less likely you are to take care of yourself: So it's important to know how much sleep you need to stay healthy—and how to make sure you get it.

SLUMBERLAND

• We all experience two kinds of sleep: REM (rapid eye movement) sleep, and non-REM sleep.

• Non-REM sleep comes first. It consists of four stages, in which sleep becomes progressively deeper, and body functions slow down until you reach your deepest sleep.

• After passing through stage 4, you enter REM sleep. Your body is limp, but your eyes twitch; heartbeat and breathing rates increase; and brainwaves become smoother. Most dreams take place during REM sleep.

• Moving through all stages of sleep takes about 90 minutes. In a good night's sleep, your body goes through the whole cycle four or five times.

• If you lose REM sleep, anxiety levels increase and you can become depressed. A lack of non-REM sleep inhibits the body's ability to heal itself and resist infections, and retards growth in children.

SIMPLE THINGS YOU CAN DO

1. Find Out What You Need

• Pick 10 average days. Keep track of the hours you sleep and how you feel during the day.

• Figure out your average amount of sleep per night for that period.

• Experts say that, in general, if you feel refreshed and can concentrate for the entire day, the average number of hours you've slept in the 10-day period is ideal for you.

2. Adjust Your Sleep Habits

• If you feel sluggish during the day, you may be sleep-deprived. Try an extra 30-90 minutes of sleep each night. But go to bed earlier instead of sleeping later. Your metabolism normally speeds up in the morning; getting up late may keep it slow, resulting in a sluggish feeling.

• If you can't get to sleep earlier than usual, catch up on sleep by taking an afternoon nap for an hour (or less) during the day. One study indicates that people who take brief naps in the afternoon are as much as 30% less likely to have heart disease.

• If you stay up late, try to get up no later than an hour from your normal time. It prevents disruption of your schedule.

3. Get Help If You Need It

• If you have insomnia, a few simple changes in environment or habits might make a difference. For example, try keeping your bedroom cool (the ideal sleeping temperature is 64°-66° F.), or avoid all forms of caffeine after noon. The resources below offer many tricks for better sleep.

• About half of people who have occasional insomnia can attribute it to stress. They recover on their own when the stress passes.

• But if things haven't improved after three weeks, talk to a doctor. You may want a referral to a sleep-disorders center for evaluation. Therapists are usually recommended for people with long-term insomnia.

RESOURCES

• **American Sleep Disorder Association**, 604 Second St., SW, Rochester, MN 55902. *Offers free brochures on all sleeping disorders and can provide a list of sleep-disorder centers and clinics in your area.*

• *No More Sleepless Nights* by Peter Hauri, Ph.D., and Shirley Linde, Ph.D. (John Wiley and Sons, 1991).

• *Sleep: Problems and Solutions* by Quentin Regestein, M.D., and David Ritchie (Consumer Reports Books, 1990).

34. BE SOCIAL

*A major California medical study showed that
social interaction may help people live longer.*

What are you doing tonight? Do you have a club meeting? A card game? A dinner party?...Or are you just staying home with your family?

Whatever you're doing, if you're planning to be with other people, you may actually be helping yourself—and them—to live longer.

SAVE YOUR LIFE
The benefits of a social network are more than just emotional:

• According to the U.S. Department of Health and Human Services, "Many of our daily conversations are actually mutual counseling sessions that help us deal with routine stresses. Scientists have found that this sort of emotional support can help prevent ill health and promotes recovery when an illness or accident occurs."

• A 10-year study by researchers at Stanford University showed that "terminally ill cancer patients who participated in weekly support group meetings, in addition to receiving treatment, lived nearly twice as long as those receiving only medical care."

• Another study found that patients with emphysema, asthma, or bronchitis had shorter periods of hospitalization after participating in self-help groups.

• Even pets can help you live longer. Research has shown that heart attack victims with pets generally live longer than those who don't have pets.

SIMPLE THINGS YOU CAN DO

1. Protect Yourself

• Spend time with friends and family. Emphasize traditions and special days—or create some of your own. Celebrate with picnics, birthday parties, family reunions, etc.

• Join clubs or social organizations. Experts say: "The most helpful contacts are regular activities that occur once a week"—such as church, community meetings, organized sports, discussion groups, etc.

• Volunteer. Any type of organization that interests you is fine, as long as your participation involves contact with other people. Just sending a check won't help you.

• Get a pet. Make sure maintenance is manageable for you. (If the pleasure doesn't outweigh the aggravation, it won't be much help.)

• Join a support group. If you have personal problems, a support group may be what you need. You'd be surprised at what you may share with other people. The ranks of the self-help groups have grown to include Compulsive Shoppers, Pedestrians First, Alcoholics Anonymous, and hundreds of others. To find out which groups meet in your community, check the yellow pages under "social service organizations," or consult your hospital, church, or temple. They may also have a community bulletin board you can consult.

RESOURCES

• **The Self-Help Clearinghouse** of the St. Clares-Riverside Medical Center, Pocono Rd, Denville, NJ 07834; (201) 625-7101. *Provides lists of groups nationwide, or guidance on setting one up in your area (for info, send a stamped, self-addressed envelope).*

• **National Self-Help Clearinghouse**, 33 West 42nd St., New York, NY 10036; (212) 642-2944.

• **California Self-Help Center**, 405 Hilgard Ave., Los Angeles, CA 90024; (213) 825-1799. *Has developed an audiotape and print program called "Common Concern." It guides groups through their formative stages, without the presence of a professional.*

• **"Plain Talk About Mutual Help Groups."** *A pamphlet from the National Institute of Mental Health, U.S. Department of Health and Human Services, 5600 Fishers Lane, Rockville, MD 20857. Includes lists of various organizations and help groups.*

35. USE MEDICINE SAFELY

*Americans down about 40 billion doses of
capsules, tablets, and liquid medications a year.*

W hen you think of dangerous drugs, you probably don't
think of medicine you can buy over the counter, or
medicine your doctor prescribes for you.

But it's estimated that every year about 300,000 people are hospitalized for the misuse of these legal medications—and about 4,000 of them die. In fact, hospital emergency rooms report that 50% of all their drug-related emergencies are due to misuse of medications.

Following a few simple guidelines can help you take the medication you need…without taking unnecessary risks at the same time.

PILLS & PERILS
Which medicines can be dangerous? Here are just a few examples:

• Diet pills containing the ingredient PPA may temporarily elevate blood pressure—a risk for people with high blood pressure.

• Medicine that's past its expiration date can be dangerous. For example, old tetracycline can cause kidney damage.

• Some drugs (e.g., Valium) increase the body's sensitivity to heat or the ultraviolet rays of the sun. So a temperature that might normally make someone sweat can cause heat stroke instead, and instead of tanning, a person might get a blistering sunburn.

• Studies show that people using tranquilizers are up to five times more likely than average to be involved in a car accident.

SIMPLE THINGS YOU CAN DO

1. Know Your Risk

• Ask your doctor for information about the proper use, possible side-effects, and abuse potential of *any* medicine you take—including over-the-counter drugs.

• Remember: Over-the-counter medicines are real drugs. Always read labels before using them, and follow directions. Taking medicine longer than recommended may hide serious medical problems.

problems.

• Your risk of having a problem with medication increases as you get older. Over time, our bodies lose the ability to process drugs efficiently, so the "adult recommended dosage" may be too strong. If you're concerned about this, discuss it with your doctor.

2. Take Precautions

• Always let your doctor know if you're taking other medications, have ever had a bad reaction to a drug, are pregnant or breast-feeding, have other illnesses, or use alcohol or tobacco. Some doctors will ask you...but some won't.

• Use one pharmacy for all your prescriptions. Interaction of two or more drugs can be harmful—even fatal. Pharmacies often have computer systems that help keep track of what you're taking. Some systems will automatically spot bad combinations of medicines prescribed by different doctors.

• Never take medicine in the dark. You might take the wrong pill if you can't see what you're taking.

• Get rid of all medicine that's past its expiration date, or doesn't have a clearly marked expiration date, any leftover antibiotics, or any medicine you don't recognize. But be careful not to put them in the garbage where children might find them.

3. Protect Your Children

• Keep medications out of children's reach, and use safety caps. If necessary, keep medicine in a locked cabinet. Note: Older adults or people without children are less likely to use safety caps and may leave medicines on counters and nightstands. One study showed that more than a third of children treated for drug misuse took the medicine at grandparents' homes.

• Never get kids to take medicine by pretending it's candy. Your child might grab a handful when you're not looking.

RESOURCES

• **The American Council for Drug Education**, 204 Monroe St., Rockville, MD, 20850; (800) 488-DRUG. *Free catalog.*

• **The National Council on Patient Education**, 666 11th St. NW, Suite 810, Washington, DC 20001; (202) 347-6711. *Write for their free pamphlet,* Get the Answers: 5 Questions Patients Should Ask When They Get a Prescription Filled. *Send a SASE envelope.*

36. COLORECTAL CANCER

*If you develop any kind of cancer, there is a
1-in-7 chance it will be colorectal cancer.*

D o you think of colorectal cancer as a "grandparent's disease"?
You're only partly right. While it's true that 90% of the cases
appear in people over 50, colorectal cancer takes many
years—sometimes more than a decade—to develop. So the
things you eat in your 30s or 40s can have a direct impact on
whether you get the disease.

The good news is that because it does develop over a period of
time, colorectal cancer can be detected long before symptoms
appear. With early detection, the survival rate is 95%. If it's not
detected early, the chances of surviving drop to less than 7%.

You can begin to protect yourself now by learning which exams
you need...and what changes you can make in your diet to mini-
mize your risk for the disease.

SAVE YOUR LIFE

• *Colorectal* is short for "colon and rectum." The colon, or large
intestine, is the last 5-6 feet of your digestive system. The last 8-10
inches of the colon is the rectum.

• This year, an estimated 112,000 Americans will be diagnosed
with colon cancer, 45,500 with rectal cancer.

• According to the American Cancer Society, early detection of
colorectal cancer through regular exams could have saved as many
as 50,000 lives last year. Instead, about 30,000 men and 30,500
women died from it—making it the second leading cause of cancer
deaths in the U.S.

SIMPLE THINGS YOU CAN DO

1. Know Your Risk

• If someone in your immediate family had colorectal cancer (or
polyps, which are small growths), you're 3 times more likely than
the average person to get it yourself.

• People living in urban, industrialized areas get colon and rectal
cancer more often than people in rural areas. No one's sure why.

• Chances of getting colon cancer appear to rise in almost direct proportion to the amount of red meat and animal fat (excluding dairy products) people eat. According to the *New England Journal of Medicine*, people who eat beef, pork or lamb every day are more than twice as likely to get colon cancer as people who avoid red meat.

• The chance of getting these diseases increases as you get older... starting at about age 40.

2. Get Tests

The American Cancer Society recommends 3 screening exams:

• After age 40: A rectal exam once a year. Purpose: It allows the doctor to feel for polyps. If polyps are found, they're removed and examined for cancer.

• After age 50: A stool blood test once a year. Purpose: It checks for hidden blood, a potential sign of cancer. Note: There's some controversy about this one. The test shows a high rate of false positives—which means, according to one expert, that people may be "needlessly subjected to invasive diagnostic tests."

• After age 60: A *proctosigmoidoscopy* once every 3-5 years. Purpose: It checks the lower 10 inches of the colon—where polyps and cancer are often found—through a hollow lighted tube.

• If you're a high-risk case, you may want to talk to your doctor about a colonoscopy. The colonoscope is a 5-foot-long tube that enables the physician to examine the entire length of the colon and remove suspicious growths. Note: This has its own slight risk. There's a small chance the instrument will perforate the bowel.

3. Protect Yourself

• Watch your diet. A high-fiber diet can protect against the disease. This means more fruit, vegetables, and whole-grain breads. (See p. 37). A recent study at Cornell found that a high-fiber, low-fat diet can actually shrink precancerous polyps.

• Cut down on the amount of red meat you eat.

RESOURCES

• National Cancer Institute; (800) 4-CANCER. *Offers free materials on colorectal cancer, including* What You Need to Know About Cancer of the Colon and Rectum.

• American Cancer Society. (800) ACS-2345. *Free materials.*

37. CHECK YOUR PROSTATE

According to the American Cancer Society, as many as one million American men have prostate cancer and don't know it.

D o you know what a prostate is? It's an important part of the male reproductive system—a walnut-sized gland, located just below the bladder, that adds fluid to semen.

Prostate cancer usually spreads without symptoms...and there are no known ways to prevent it. So early detection through regular screening tests is the key to survival.

SAVE YOUR LIFE

• Early detection makes the difference. Despite the fact that 85% of localized cases can be cured in the early stages, an estimated 32,000 men will die this year because of prostate cancer.

• Prostate cancer is commonly considered an "old man's disease," but one out of five cases occurs in men younger than 65.

• One in eleven men will develop prostate cancer.

SIMPLE THINGS YOU CAN DO

Get Tested

• A rectal exam is "a quick, painless procedure in which the doctor inserts a gloved finger and presses against the prostate to feel for tumors." Men over 40 should get one every year.

• Your doctor may also recommend a blood test. Ask about it.

RESOURCES

• The National Cancer Institute, (800) 4-CANCER; American Cancer Society, (800) ACS-2345. *Both offer free materials. Ask for NCI's* What You Need to Know About Prostate Cancer.

• Patient Advocates for Advanced Cancer Treatment, 1143 Parmelee NW, Grand Rapids, MI 49504; (616) 453-1477. *Provides free information on prostate cancer treatment options.*

38. DO A HOME SAFETY AUDIT

Every ten seconds, an American is injured at home.

Did you know that you're more likely to have an accident at home than anywhere else? Every year, about 4 million Americans are disabled in home accidents...and about 20,000 of them die.

Of course, no home can be made 100% accident-proof. But there are things you can do to reduce the possibility of a serious accident happening in *your* home. As a first step, the National Safety Council recommends a room-by-room "safety audit."

SAVE YOUR LIFE
• The most common fatal home accidents are falls. In 1990, for example, more than 1 million people were admitted to emergency rooms after falling down stairs. Many of these accidents could have been prevented if light switches were installed at the top and bottom of the stairways.

• Burns are a danger, especially to children. Turning your water heater down to 120° can prevent scalding.

• About 500 people are electrocuted at home every year. Installing "ground fault circuit interrupter outlets" can help prevent shocks.

SIMPLE THINGS YOU CAN DO
1. Know What to Look For
• Send for the National Safety Council's booklet, "Home Safety." It provides a checklist of potential safety problems to look for around your home...and tells you how to correct them.

• Write to: National Safety Council, 444 North Michigan Ave., Chicago, IL 60611.

2. Protect Yourself
• Make a list of the changes you need to make.

• Make the easy ones right away, and set time aside for the more involved projects.

39. PREVENT FALLS

Falls are the leading cause of accidental deaths among seniors.

If you're young and you slip and fall, you might feel a little sore... but you'll probably recover easily.

But if you're an older person, falling down could mean broken bones, internal injuries...or even death. Fortunately, most falls can be prevented by taking a few simple precautions.

SAVE YOUR LIFE

• About 9,000 people die each year from falls or related injuries. About 75% of these people are over 65.

• Many falls appear to cause nothing worse than a bruise. But older people have fragile skin and small blood vessels that make bruising more serious. Even a gentle blow to the head can cause dangerous delayed bleeding within the skull.

• Many older people fall and can't get back up, even though they're not seriously injured. If they lie on a cold floor for hours before getting help, it can lead to hypothermia (low body temperature) and pneumonia.

• Even if an older person is not badly injured, falling can make them frightened and less confident. As a result, many older people become less active after a fall, which only makes them weaker and more prone to other accidents.

SIMPLE THINGS YOU CAN DO

1. Know Your Risk

• As we get older, our bones become weaker. Women especially lose bone strength because they lose calcium after menopause, a condition known as *osteoporosis*. This is why it's common for senior citizens to "break their hips" when they fall. Actually, it's not the hip, but the top of the femur, or thigh bone, that's broken.

• The incidence of so-called "broken hips" doubles about every seven years after the age of 65. By the age of 90, one woman in four has suffered this type of fracture.

2. Take Precautions

• Check your home for hazards that could cause a fall. (See p. 73).

• Keep a flashlight or lamp next to the bed, so you won't risk tripping in the dark; or use a night light.

• Store clothes and other items where you can reach them without standing on a stool or chair. If you need something that's out of your reach, wait and have someone else get it down for you.

• Slip-proof your shower and tubs by placing non-skid mats or abrasive strips on slick surfaces. Also use a non-skid mat next to the tub, or cover the floor with carpet. Install handrails in and near baths.

• Keep all stairways well lit, with a switch at top and bottom.

• Make sure that all carpets are securely attached to the floor.

• Install handrails or banisters along all indoor and outdoor steps. As many as 2.6 million people are hurt each year climbing stairs.

3. Get Help If You Need It

• If you live alone, work out a way of alerting others if you have an accident. For example, carry a whistle to blow if you fall down and can't get back up. Or schedule regular phone calls with family and friends. If the schedule is disrupted, they'll know to check on you.

• If you fall and are in pain, see your doctor. According to the AMA, "It is important to relieve the pain as quickly as possible so a person can keep moving. Bed may seem to be the most comfortable place, but it is too easy for someone who is already stiff and sore after a fall to become bedbound and immobile."

4. Exercise

• Much of the physical frailty attributed to aging is actually due to a lack of exercise. It's never too late. According to some experts, even if you've been inactive for a long time, a moderate exercise program can "stimulate the formation of new bone tissue, and improve cardiovascular endurance, muscle strength, and flexibility." Note: Be sure to consult a physician before starting a new exercise program.

RESOURCES

• **American Association of Retired Persons (AARP),** *601 E Street, NW, Washington DC 20049. Offers hundreds of free pamphlets, including* Pep Up Your Life: A Fitness Book for Seniors. *Write for membership information.*

40. HAVE AN EMERGENCY FIRE ESCAPE PLAN

Smoke inhalation is responsible for 80% of all fire deaths.

Every year, home fires in the U.S. claim more than 4,000 lives and injure at least 250,000 people. Most of these deaths occur between 10 p.m. and 6 a.m., when people are sleeping.

The only way you can be sure your family will know what to do if they wake up to a fire is to have an emergency escape plan, and to practice regular fire drills in your home.

SIMPLE THINGS YOU CAN DO

Have an Escape Plan

• Make sure everyone in your family knows what your smoke detector alarm sounds like and how to respond to it.

• With your family, draw a simple floor plan of your home, showing all possible exits. Pick two exits from each room, in case one is blocked. Keep these exits clear of obstructions at all times.

• If necessary, buy rope or chain ladders to use for climbing out of windows above the first floor. Keep them near the window.

• Have a designated meeting place outside the house, preferably in front where firefighters can see you so they'll know you aren't trapped.

• If you live in an apartment or condominium, know how to get to the exit stairs. Never take an elevator; in a fire, an elevator shaft is like a smokestack; an elevator will quickly fill up with smoke.

• Have a regular fire drill, and practice how to escape.

• There are many more important details to learn. Ask your local Red Cross for the free flyer, "Are Your Ready for a Fire?" or contact the NFPA (below) for more information.

RESOURCES

• **National Fire Protection Association Public Affairs Office,** Dept. TFH, PO Box 9146, 1 Batterymarch Park, Quincy, MA 02269, (800) 344-3555. *Call for a free catalog of fire safety and prevention materials (including comic books for educating kids).*

IT TAKES A

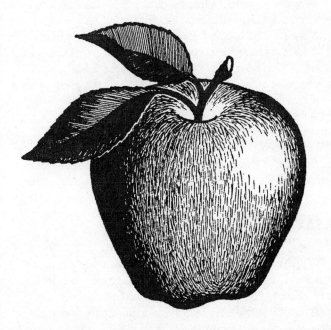

COMMITMENT

41. LEARN CPR

*About 100,000 lives are saved each year by
people who have learned CPR.*

One morning, while he was brushing his teeth, 48-year-old Frank Gerow had a heart attack. His 17-year-old son, Pete, heard a crash and rushed upstairs to find his father unconscious on the bathroom floor. Pete had just been trained in CPR (*cardiopulmonary resuscitation*). "I knew what had to be done, and I just did it," he recalls. Pete saved his father's life.

He's not alone. Since CPR was introduced about thirty years ago, the percentage of heart attack victims who make it to the hospital for treatment has risen from 5% to 25%.

According to the American Heart Association, about half a million Americans will die from coronary artery disease this year. At least one-third of them could survive if they receive immediate emergency (CPR or ambulance) care. By taking the time to learn CPR, you can save a life, too.

CPR SAVES LIVES
Proof that CPR can make a difference:
• In 1971, the city of Seattle, Washington, launched a program to train citizens in CPR. First, firefighters were trained as CPR instructors. Then, a 3-hour course was offered free to the public. CPR training became mandatory for 9th- and 10th-grade students.

• So far, more than 400,000 people in Seattle have been trained in CPR, and 2,000 more take the course every month. About one out of every three residents now knows CPR.

• Before the training program began, only 5% of heart attack victims in Seattle were given CPR by a bystander. After the first 10 years of community-wide training, this figure increased to 40%—and the survival rate doubled.

HOW DOES CPR WORK?
We can't teach you CPR in a book, but here's an idea of what it does:
• When someone's heart and breathing stop, it can take only four

to eight minutes before the victim suffers brain damage and dies. CPR buys precious time by keeping blood and oxygen circulating through the victim's body until they can be resuscitated.

- People trained in CPR learn the ABCs of saving lives:

Airway: Tilt the victim's head back to clear an airway.

Breathing: Pinch the nose and perform mouth-to-mouth rescue breathing.

Circulation: Use both hands to compress the victim's chest so the heart delivers blood to the body.

- CPR can't "restart" someone's heart. The heartbeat is triggered by an electrical impulse, and when it stops it can only be started again by another electrical impulse—such as the "shock paddles" you've probably seen on TV. But CPR increases the chances that the victim will have a chance to be resuscitated this way. It artificially keeps circulation going until paramedics arrive.

SIMPLE THINGS YOU CAN DO

1. Take a CPR Course
You can take one through the Red Cross, YMCA, or other organization. It's easy to learn; most adults and children over 12 can do it. In fact, more than 50 million Americans have been trained in CPR; and about 5 million take CPR courses each year. Courses cost about $30 and take about 3 hours. You'll learn how to handle a number of emergency situations, including near drownings, heart attacks, and chokings.

2. Take a Refresher Course
If you already know CPR, but haven't taken a course in a few years, it's good to brush up on your life-saving skills. Some of the techniques have been changed and improved.

RESOURCES

- **American Red Cross**, 17th and D St. NW, Washington, DC 20006. *Contact a local chapter or write for "CPR Saves Lives." Free.*

- **National Safety Council**, 444 N. Michigan Ave., Chicago, IL 60611. *Write for a free copy of "Pocket Guide to First Aid."*

- **American Heart Association.** *Contact your local chapter for a pamphlet on CPR and a CPR Wall Chart. Cost is 25¢.*

42. REDUCE RADON

Radon, a naturally occurring gas, accounts for more than half of the American public's total exposure to harmful radiation.

I n December 1984, an engineer named Stanley Watras set off radiation alarms as he walked into work at the Limerick nuclear power station. Since he'd just arrived, he obviously hadn't been contaminated at the plant. So where did the radiation come from?

The source turned out to be radon gas coming from the ground under his home. The level was so high that his health risk was equal to smoking more than 100 packs of cigarettes a day. The Watras family was evacuated while contractors eliminated the problem...and Americans became aware of radon for the first time.

Today, the EPA considers radon a major health risk; potentially dangerous levels of the gas have been found in homes in every state. However, there's no need to panic; even homes with high radon levels can be made safe with minor modifications. The important first step is to get your home tested to see if you have radon problems.

THE RADON REPORT

• Radon is an invisible, odorless, tasteless gas that's created when uranium in rock and soil decays. It quickly dissipates in the open air...but in a house, it can collect in dangerous concentrations.

• Why is it dangerous? If it's breathed in, it can disintegrate and leave radioactive byproducts in a person's lungs. These substances can lodge there and cause cancer.

• According to the Surgeon General, radon gas is the second-biggest cause of lung cancer in the U.S., after smoking.

• Radon-exposed smokers or former smokers are up to ten times more likely than people who never smoked to get radon-induced lung cancer

• The EPA reports that radon causes about 14,000 deaths a year.

• The EPA and the Public Health Service estimate that 8 million U.S. homes contain unsafe levels of radon, yet 95% of U.S. homes haven't even been tested.

SIMPLE THINGS YOU CAN DO

1. Know Your Risk

• The only accurate way to tell whether a home contains radon is to test for it. The EPA and U.S. Surgeon General recommend that everyone living in a detached house, town house, or apartment in the basement or on the second or first floor test for it.

2. Know What to Look For

• If you have a professional come in and check your radon level, make sure they've completed the EPA's most recent Radon Proficiency Program. Your state radon office should have a list of qualified companies in your area.

• Some utilities offer the test for free as part of an energy audit.

• You can do it yourself. Pick up an EPA-approved short-term radon detector at a hardware store. (Some experts suggest the charcoal canister type). Follow directions carefully. Leave the detector in place for the specified amount of time. Then send it to the manufacturer for a reading. Expect to pay $12-$26 for the canister, laboratory fee, and report.

• Wait 2 weeks for the lab results. If the reading is high, the EPA recommends a second test. If you still get a high reading, your home may need modifications.

3. Protect Yourself

• Reduce the radon. This can be done in a number of ways, from sealing basement cracks to installing a ventilation system under the house foundation. You may need a contractor for the job. State environmental protection departments and the EPA can provide a list of approved contractors able to make these modifications.

• If you're buying a home, ask if the house has been checked for radon. If not, get the test done before proceeding.

RESOURCES

• **EPA, Center for Environmental Research Information**, 26 W. Martin Luther King Dr., Cincinnati, OH 45268. *Request their free booklets on radon, including* Radon Reduction Methods. Call (800) SOS-RADON for information.

• **American Lung Association.** *Call your local chapter for info.*

43. LIGHTEN UP

*In 1990, Americans spent an estimated $36 billion on
diets and diet-related products and services.*

How's your weight? Could you afford to lose a few pounds? Studies show that obese people are at greater risk for certain kinds of cancer, heart disease, strokes, high blood pressure and diabetes.

But it's not just the seriously overweight who need to watch the scales. Even if you're carrying an extra 10 pounds, it could be affecting your health.

SAVE YOUR LIFE

• It's estimated that one in five Americans is obese—i.e, at least 20% above their desirable weight due to excess body fat. In some cases, the extra weight is due partly to genetics, but overeating and lack of exercise are the most common culprits.

• According to the 1988 Surgeon General's Report on Nutrition and Health, being 20% overweight can lower a woman's life expectancy by 10% and a man's by 20%.

• However, recent studies show that weight losses of even 10-25 pounds may help obese people reduce health hazards like high blood pressure and low blood sugar.

ABOUT DIETING

• 48 million Americans are currently on a diet. But dieting often doesn't work. People who lose weight rapidly are three times more likely to regain it than those who take pounds off more slowly.

• Dieting can have unexpected results: The first pounds lost in a diet are water. If a dieter doesn't excercise, the next few pounds lost are muscle—sometimes even heart muscle. When muscle is gone, the body needs less energy, so more food is turned into fat. Dieters who excercise don't lose muscle.

• Losing/gaining weight over and over again is called "yo-yo dieting." It not only makes weight control tough, but may threaten your life. The Framingham Heart Study found that people whose weight shifted the most during the 14-year study had about a 50% higher risk for heart disease than people whose weight was stable.

SIMPLE THINGS YOU CAN DO

1. Know What to Look For

• If you're not sure whether you're overweight, contact your doctor or another health professional to discuss it.

• Where your fat is located may be more important than how much you've got. Recent evidence suggests that "apple-shaped" people, whose fat is concentrated in the abdomen (e.g., people with beer-bellies) may have a greater risk of cardiovascular disease than "pear-shaped" people with fat around the hips and buttocks.

• Be realistic. If you're dieting correctly, you can't expect to lose thirty pounds in a month; aim for smaller, short-term goals, like one or two pounds a week.

2. Protect Yourself

• Go for a permanent weight reduction by making your weight-loss program a lifestyle change…instead of a diet.

√ Exercise. It's an essential part of keeping weight off. Nevertheless, Americans have reduced their physical activity by an estimated 75% since 1900. (See pp. 20, 24, 38 for more information on exercise.)

√ Eat moderately and sensibly. To lose a pound a week, you need to eat 500 fewer calories a day. Ways to reduce calories: Eat more complex carbohydrates and less fat; snack on fruits and vegetables instead of junk food. (For more information, contact the Resources below.)

RESOURCES

• **The American Dietetic Association**, 216 W. Jackson Blvd., Chicago, IL 60606-6995. *Write for a free catalog that contains over 50 brochures and books including* Why Can't I Lose Weight *and* Weight Expectations: Weight Loss and You.

• **The Weight Maintenance Survival Guide**, *by Judith Rodin and Kelly Brownell (American Health Publishing Co., 1990). Based on research on dieting and weight control, this book contains the most successful weight maintenance strategies.*

44. COPING WITH STRESS

According to the American Council of Family Physicians, approximately two-thirds of all visits to family doctors are for stress-related disorders.

Nobody has to tell you what stress is. You already know. The question is: How are you handling it?...And what can you do about it?

ABOUT STRESS

• Stress isn't intrinsically good or bad. It's how you *perceive* a situation that makes stress good or bad—not the situation itself. Some commuters, for instance, don't mind traffic; others become enraged by it. "The significance of this," says a recent report, "is that if you can control your *view* of events, even if you can't control events themselves, you can control stress."

• Many researchers believe stress comes from a primitive physiological response to a perceived threat or danger—a "fight or flight" reaction. Your body gets ready to do battle or run away...but there's no physical release. "Most people don't punch the boss or race out of the office screaming, even though their bodies may be primed to do so," explains one expert. "Instead, they may develop psychiatric symptoms, a tension headache, or abdominal pains."

• "When the 'fight or flight response' becomes chronic, as it does in battle, longterm chemical changes occur, leading to high blood pressure, an increased rate of atherosclerosis, depression of the immune system, and other problems."

• When you're under stress, hormones like *cortisol* and *epinepherine* are released. Both hormones can raise blood pressure and cortisol can depress the immune system.

SIMPLE THINGS YOU CAN DO

1. Protect Yourself

• Learn to recognize your stress symptoms, and be prepared to deal with them.

• Talk to people. There's growing evidence that social support can help you weather stressful times (see p. 66). Talking to a friend, family member, or counselor can also help you recognize what's bothering you.

• Getting regular exercise (see p. 24), eating a balanced diet (p. 32), and getting enough sleep (p. 64), can reduce stress.

• Eliminate as many stress sources as you can—for example, try turning the TV off to stop noise. Or clean up a cluttered area.

• Sometimes you can't get rid of stress in your environment—so you have to leave your environment. Learn how to get away for a while. Take a walk, use relaxation techniques (see below).

2. Plan Ahead.

• Manage your time. It's important to realize you can't do everything. Make a list of the things you have to do, in order of importance. Once you see them on paper, it may be apparent you're trying to do too much.

• Learn to say no to things you really don't want to do.

• Avoid predictably stressful situations like driving in rush hour, or socializing with people you don't like.

• Learn to relax. If you teach yourself how to relax when you're not tense, you can use it when you are. Here's one easy technique:

√ Find a quiet place, get in a comfortable position, inhale/exhale deeply twice.

√ Tense, then relax the muscles in each part of your body (e.g., forehead, neck, hands, arms, abdomen, legs), one body part at a time, going from head to toe. Inhale/exhale after relaxing each body part.

√ When you're relaxed down to your toes, inhale and exhale twice while thinking the word *One* or *Relax*.

√ Practice every day for two weeks, then practice about once or twice a week thereafter.

√ When you're feeling stress, inhale/exhale while thinking your chosen word (Step 3). If you're experiencing tension in a particular body part, tense and relax that muscle group.

RESOURCES

The American Institute of Stress, 124 Park Ave., Yonkers, NY 10703; (914) 963-1200. *Send a SASE for information.*

45. QUIT SMOKING

Every two seconds, an American permanently gives up smoking.

Anyone who's ever smoked knows how difficult it is to quit. Some people try and fail over and over. But according to the Harvard Medical School, the more times you try, the more likely you are to succeed. And the good news is that when you finally quit, your body begins repairing itself right away. After a year of not smoking, for instance, your risk of tobacco-related heart disease will be reduced by 50%, and in a few years, your risk of cardiac problems will be the same as if you'd never smoked at all.

This year, more than 1.3 million people will give up smoking for good. You can be one of them.

HOLY SMOKE!

• Fifty million Americans smoke 1.6 billion cigarettes a day.

• According to a Gallup poll, about 80% of smokers say they'd like to quit. And many are succeeding. 38 million Americans—nearly half of all living adults who've ever smoked—have quit smoking.

• One reason quitting is so hard: Nicotine (a substance present only in the tobacco leaf). The Surgeon General has found nicotine to be as addictive as heroin or cocaine.

• Over 434,000 Americans die prematurely each year from the effects of tobacco.

• Cigarette smoke contains more than 40 carcinogens.

SECOND-HAND SMOKE

• Smoking isn't just an issue of individual freedom. It affects non-smokers, too. According to the American Heart Association, second-hand smoke (the smoke from other people's cigarettes) is the third-largest preventable cause of death in the U.S., taking about 54,000 lives a year.

• Reports show that the unfiltered smoke that comes off the burning end of a cigarette "actually contains higher amounts of the compounds that cause cancer and heart disease than what the smoker inhales."

SIMPLE THINGS YOU CAN DO

1. Know Your Risk

• Smokers are ten times as likely to get lung cancer, and three times as likely to die of strokes as non-smokers.

• "Light" cigarettes don't reduce heart attack risk. A recent study showed smokers were four times more likely to have a first heart attack than nonsmokers, no matter what brand they smoked.

• You might think you'll gain a lot of weight if you quit, but the average quitter gains just 5 pounds. Doctors agree that gaining the average 5 pounds is no big deal compared to the risks of continued smoking.

2. Know What to Look For

• See what stop-smoking programs are available in your area. Call the local American Cancer Society, American Heart Association or American Lung Association. (They have a variety of programs.) Many hospitals and health maintenance organizations (HMOs) also offer programs or can supply referrals to other programs.

• Look into the wide variety of quitting methods, including self-help books, hypnosis, nicotine gum and nicotine patches (prescribed by a doctor or dentist), support groups, acupuncture, etc.

3. Plan Ahead

• After you've done some research, list the various programs or methods that appeal to you. Experts say this is important, because:

√ Different methods work for different people.

√ You may have to try a number of programs before you find one that works.

√ Studies show that a person is more likely to give up an addiction if there are several options to choose from.

• Keep trying until you find the method that works for you.

RESOURCES

• **The American Cancer Society,** 1599 Clifton Road NE, Atlanta, GA 30329; (800) ACS-2345.

• **The American Lung Association,** 1740 Broadway, New York, NY 10019-4374; (212) 315-8700.

46. SUBSTANCE ABUSE

Forty percent of Americans do not drink at all. Of those who do drink, about ten percent account for half of all the alcohol consumed.

Here's a sobering thought: More than 20 million Americans are addicted to alcohol or other drugs...and more than 100,000 of them will suffer drug- or alcohol-related deaths this year. Unfortunately, many people with substance abuse problems don't realize it. As their lives slowly deteriorate, they fail to understand the cause—or that they need help.

Could you, or someone you love, be one of these people?

Recovering from addiction is never easy, but people don't have to do it alone. There are organizations in every community to which people can turn. They've helped hundreds of thousands of Americans recover from addictions. They can help you, too.

SAVE YOUR LIFE

• Alcoholism is a progressive disease that is characterized by a gradual increase in tolerance and a gradual deterioration in lifestyle. Some 18 million Americans are either alcoholics or alcohol abusers—one out of every ten adults.

• The American Council on Alcoholism reports that excessive drinking can shorten a person's life span by 10-12 years. Abusing alcohol over a long period of time can cause liver damage, heart disease, ulcers, cancer of the mouth, stomach and esophagus, and even brain damage.

• Pregnant women who drink excessively risk having a child with fetal alcohol syndrome, the third leading cause of mental retardation. Even women who drink small amounts of alcohol during pregnancy— just one or two drink a day— increase their risk of having a baby with some of the effects of fetal alcohol syndrome, including a lower birth weight.

• Marijuana may seem harmless, but extensive use can damage your body's respiratory, reproductive, cardiovascular, and nervous systems. And one marijuana cigarette contains more cancer-causing agents than a regular cigarette.

• Cocaine use constricts blood vessels and increases your heartbeat when it enters your body; large doses can cause palpitations, erratic heartbeats, convulsions, and even death.

SIMPLE THINGS YOU CAN DO

1. Know What to Look For

• Here are some warning signs of drug or alcohol dependency:

√ A regular habit that's becoming hard to control.

√ A substantial increase in drug or alcohol tolerance over time.

√ Trouble with your family, at work, or with the law, because of drinking or drugs.

√ Blackouts.

√ Repeatedly trying to quit unsuccessfully.

√ An inability to limit the amount of drugs or alcohol you consume. You can't consistently predict when and if you're going to start...and once you've started, you can't predict when—or if—you're going to stop.

• If you've experienced more than one or two of these symptoms, chances are you have a substance abuse problem. Note: These are major symptoms. There are many others. If you even wonder whether you have a substance abuse problem, that may be a symptom.

2. Get Help if You Need it.

• There are many drug treatment options available, including group therapy, psychiatric counseling, and detoxification centers. The treatment that's right for you depend on the extent of your illness. Treatment for chemical dependency is often covered by medical insurance.

RESOURCES

• Alcoholics Anonymous, P.O. Box 459, Grand Central Station, New York, NY 10163; (212) 686-1100 or call a local AA office.

• National Council on Alcoholism and Drug Dependence, 12 West 21st Street, New York, NY 10010; (800) NCA-CALL.

• National Institute on Drug Abuse Helpline; (800) 843-4971; Information resource for alcohol and drug problems.

47. LAUGHING MATTERS

Studies have shown that "a 4-year-old child laughs up to 500 times a day. An adult, on average, laughs only 15 times a day."

You probably don't think of laughter as medicine...but a number of doctors now believe it can help people live longer. One specialist calls it "inner jogging."

Norman Cousins, who introduced the idea of "laughter therapy" in the late '70s, noted: "In the few years that humor has become an area of medical interest, researchers have detailed a wide array of beneficial changes brought about by laughter—everything from enhanced respiration to increased immune-cell activity."

THE BEST MEDICINE

• According to William Fry, Jr. of the Stanford Medical School, "Laughing 100 times a day is the cardiovascular equivalent of rowing for 10 minutes."

• A study conducted by Dr. Kathleen Dillon shows that "people who use humor as a coping device in everyday life" have higher levels of infection-fighting antibodies. Her conclusion: "The benefits of laughter may be cumulative, like the benefits of exercise."

• A 1989 study at Duke University found that laughter may prevent heart attacks by defusing anger.

SIMPLE THINGS YOU CAN DO

Start Today

• Figure out what makes you laugh...and put more of it in your life.

• Keep a "humor first-aid kit" around— books, cartoons, tapes, funny masks and glasses, and toys you can pull out when you need a laugh.

• Take a regular "humor break" every day.

RESOURCE

The HUMOR Project, 10 Spring St., Saratoga Springs, NY 12866. *They publish a quarterly called* Laughing Matters, *about using humor for good health. For details, send a self-addressed 9x12-inch envelope with 75¢ postage.*

48. IS IT JUST THE BLUES?

*Depression is one of the most common mental illness in the United States.
It's estimated that about 10% of all women and 5% of all men
in America will experience some symptoms of clinical depression.*

E veryone feels "down" occasionally. It's normal, for example,
to become sad or discouraged when we go through difficult
times, or to grieve when we lose something of value.

But serious depression—what doctors call "major" or "clinical"
depression—is another matter. People who are clinically depressed
sometimes feel down for months, even years. They may be unable
to work or function normally—even to eat or get out of bed. And
they might feel hopeless and out of control, as if things can never
get better.

But things *can* get better...with treatment.

Learning to recognize the symptoms of clinical depression means
you—or someone you care about—can get help when it's needed.

THE GREAT DEPRESSION

• According to the American Psychiatric Association, 80-90% of
people who are depressed can be treated effectively. However,
many people suffering from depression don't realize they have an
illness...so they never seek treatment.

• Depressed people are often more susceptible to illness because
they often don't eat right, exercise, etc.

• But the biggest danger may be suicide...the eighth-leading cause
of death in America. According to the National Institute for
Mental Health, in one study, clinically depressed people had a rate
of suicide 25 times higher than the general population.

SIMPLE THINGS YOU CAN DO

1. Know Your Risk

• Major depression can happen to anyone, and it can be brought
on by a wide variety of circumstances, from the death of a loved
one...to losing a job...to a physical condition. Depression can also
be a side effect of some illnesses.

• Genetic factors may make some people more susceptible to depression. Environmental factors may play a role, too.

2. Know What to Look For

• If you're depressed, you might not know it. That's why it's important to recognize the symptoms. If four or more of these symptoms last continually for more than two weeks, seek help:

√ Pervasive feelings of sadness, helplessness, guilt and irritability.

√ Gaining or (more often) losing a lot of weight without dieting.

√ A change in sleeping patterns. Insomnia, especially waking up too early in the morning, may be a tell-tale sign of depression.

√ Difficulty in concentrating or making decisions.

√ Loss of interest in activities you used to enjoy (including sex). You may feel withdrawn and prefer to be alone more than usual.

√ Hopelessness and/or suicidal thoughts.

√ Loss of energy; fatigue.

√ Outbursts of crying for no evident reason.

3. Get Help If You Need It

• The most important thing to do if you're depressed is to get appropriate professional help.

• To find a qualified therapist, call a doctor, a local psychological or psychiatric society, a community mental health center, or an HMO for referrals. Ask for the names of 2 or 3 people to call. Many therapists charge on a sliding scale, depending on ability to pay.

• Relieving depression may take some time, but treatment is almost always of some benefit. In most cases you'll be given therapy, medication, or a combination of both.

RESOURCES

• **National Institute of Mental Health.** D/ART, 5600 Fishers Lane, Room 10-85, Rockville, MD 20857; (800) 421-4211 (for free brochures).

• **National Mental Health Association,** 1021 Prince Street, Alexandria, VA 22314; (800) 969-NMHA.

• **Suicide & Crisis Hotline.** National toll free numbers: (800) 333-4444, (800)448-8888. *Operates 24 hours a day.*

49. A SECOND OPINION

Experts estimate that 1 of every 5 operations
performed in the U.S. is unnecessary.

W hat would you do if your doctor said you needed major
surgery? Would you just accept that opinion, because the
doctor "knows more than you do"?

That could be a mistake; surgery is always a risk...and doctors
are only human. To be sure you really need an operation, it's best
to get a second opinion.

OPERATING PROCEDURE

• About 80% of all surgery performed in the U.S. is elective (not
an emergency). The patient has time to decide when and where to
have the surgery...or whether to have it at all. If you use that time
to get a second opinion, experts estimate you'll find a better
alternative from 20% to 35% of the time.

• Some people think getting a second opinion will offend their
doctor. It won't. It's a routine part of medical procedure.

• Second opinions are often covered completely by health insurance, including Medicare and Medicaid. In fact, insurance
companies often require second opinions before elective surgery.

SIMPLE THINGS YOU CAN DO

1. Know What to Look For

• Get referrals. Ask your doctor or a hospital (preferably a teaching
hospital or medical school) for names of recommended specialists.

• Consult the book *How to Get a Second Opinion*, by Isadore Rosenfeld (Ballantine Books, 1981). It's the best resource available.

2. Protect Yourself

• Get a second opinion if you feel a diagnosis needs confirmation,
major surgery is recommended, you don't have confidence in your
doctor, or you feel dissatisfied with the progress you're making.

• Tell your doctor that you're getting a second opinion.

• If there's a conflict, get a third, even a fourth opinion. But be-
ware of shopping around for what you want to hear.

50. SHAKE, RATTLE, & ROLL

Every year, some 80 hurricanes and 100 powerful earthquakes strike worldwide...and 850 tornadoes strike in the U.S. alone.

I f you heard a report that a hurricane was coming, would you know what to do? If you saw a tornado in the distance, where would you go? A natural disaster may never happen in your area—but if it does, preparing for it now could save your and your family's lives.

SIMPLE THINGS YOU CAN DO

1. Know Your Risk

• Call your local Red Cross to find out if your area is affected by natural disasters.

2. Plan Ahead

• Create a family emergency plan. If you live in an area affected by floods or hurricanes, plan where you'll go if you're told to evacuate. If you live in an area affected by tornadoes or earthquakes, practice a tornado or earthquake safety drill. Call your local Red Cross for details.

• Decide on a central place for your family to meet following a disaster, in case you're not together when it strikes.

• Pick a contact person. Everyone in your family should memorize the phone number of a person in another state (or outside the area) to contact following a disaster. It may be the only way family members can communicate with each other.

• Find out about other emergency plans. Learn about the emergency plans at your workplace and at your children's daycare center or schools.

RESOURCES

• *The Family Survival Guide.* A comprehensive booklet from the American Red Cross about preparing for many types of disasters. Includes detailed information about first aid and emergency supplies. Contact your local chapter and ask for it. (Stock number 329195).

RECOMMENDED READING

JOURNALS AND NEWSLETTERS

Harvard Health Letter, P.O. Box 420300, Palm Coast, FL 32142-0300. $24/yr. - 12 issues

Mayo Clinic Health Letter, Subscription Services, P.O. Box 53889, Boulder, CO 80322-3889. $24-yr. - 12 issues

U.C. Berkeley Wellness Letter, Subscription Dept., P.O. Box 420148, Palm Coast, FL 32142. $24-yr. - 12 issues

Edell Health Letter, P.O. Box 57812, Boulder, CO 80322-7812. $24/yr. - 10 issues

HealthFacts, The Center for Medical Consumers, 237 Thompson St., New York, NY 10012. $21/yr. - 12 issues

New England Journal of Medicine, P.O. Box 9140, Waltham, MA 02254-9881. $89/yr. - 52 issues

Journal of the American Medical Association (JAMA) Subscription Dept., American Medical Association, 515 N. State St., Chicago, IL 60610-9802. $79/yr. - 12 issues

REFERENCE BOOKS

A small selection of the many fine books available:

Mayo Clinic Family Health Book, Mayo Foundation for Medical Education and Research. William Morrow and Co., 1990

The Wellness Encyclopedia, University of California, Berkeley, Health Letter Associates, Houghton Mifflin Co., 1991.

The American Medical Association Handbook of First Aid and Emergency Care, Random House, 1990.

The American Medical Association Family Medical Guide, Random House, 1987.

Home Medical Guide, The Columbia University College of

Physicians and Surgeons, Crown Books, 1989

The Tufts University Guide to Total Nutrition, Harpers Perennial, 1990

Prevention's Giant Book of Health Facts, Editors of Prevention Magazine, Rodale Press, 1991

Jane Brody's Nutrition Book: A Lifetime Guide to Good Eating for Better Health and Weight Control. Bantam, 1988

Guide to Personal Health, Jane Brody, Avon Books, 1976

Modern Prevention, Isadore Rosenfeld, M.D. Bantam, 1991

The Complete Guide to Living with High Blood Pressure Michael D. Rees, M.D., Consumer Reports Books, 1988

Make Sure You Do Not Have Breast Cancer Philip Strax, M.D., St. Martin's Press, 1989

Strokes: What Families Should Know, Elaine Fantle Shimberg. Ballantine Books, 1990

Cancer: The Complete Book of Cancer Prevention, Editors of Prevention Magazine Health Books. Rodale Press, 1988

The Complete Guide to Women's Health, Bruce D. Shephard M.D., F.A.C.O.G. and Carroll A. Shephard, R.N., Ph.D., Plume, 1990.

Dr. Heimlich's Home Guide to Emergency Medical Situations, Henry J. Heimlich, M.D. and Lawrence Galton, Simon and Schuster, 1980.

Take Care of Yourself, Donald M. Vickery, M.D. and James F. Fries, M.D. Addison Wesley, 1989.

The Prostate Book: Sound Advice on Symptoms and Treatment, Stephen N. Roud, M.D., Consumer Reports Books, 1988.

The American Cancer Society's "Freshstart:" 21 Days to Stop Smoking. Pocket Books, 1986.

Your Good Health: How to Stay Well and What to Do When You're Not, Harvard Medical School. Harvard University Press, 1987.